Care Trusts: Partnership Working in Action

Edited by

Jon Glasby

Lecturer
Health Services Management Centre
University of Birmingham

and

Edward Peck

Professor of Healthcare Partnerships
Director, Health Services Management Centre
University of Birmingham

Radcliffe Medical Press

Radcliffe Medical Press Ltd
18 Marcham Road
Abingdon
Oxon OX14 1AA
United Kingdom

www.radcliffe-oxford.com
The Radcliffe Medical Press electronic catalogue and online ordering facility.
Direct sales to anywhere in the world.

British Library Cataloguing in Publication Data

A catalogue record for this book is available from the British Library.

ISBN 1 85775 821 8

Typeset by Advance Typesetting Ltd, Oxfordshire
Printed and bound by TJ International Ltd, Padstow, Cornwall

Contents

List of contributors

Diane Brodie, Mental health service user, South Somerset MIND

Terry Butler, Director of Social Services, Hampshire

Shane Giles, Department of Health Care Trusts Project Manager (2001/02) and currently Director of the Integrated Care Network

Dr Jon Glasby, Lecturer, Health Services Management Centre, University of Birmingham

Professor Caroline Glendinning, Professor of Social Policy, National Primary Care Research and Development Centre, University of Manchester

Dr Nick Goodwin, Lecturer, Health Services Management Centre, University of Birmingham

Pauline Gulliver, Research Fellow, University of Otago, New Zealand

Brian Hardy, Principal Research Fellow, Nuffield Institute for Health, University of Leeds

Bob Hudson, Senior Associate, Health Services Management Centre, University of Birmingham

Angela Jeffrey, Chief Executive, New Forest Primary Care Trust

Lotta Macfarlane, Project Manager, Sandwell Mental Health NHS and Social Care Trust

Lucy O'Leary, Head of Organisational Development, Northumberland Care Trust

Professor Edward Peck, Professor of Healthcare Partnerships and Director, Health Services Management Centre, University of Birmingham

Sue Peet, Research Fellow, Nuffield Community Care Studies Unit, University of Leicester

Richard Poxton, Independent Health and Social Care Development Consultant

David Towell, Senior Research Fellow, Institute for Applied Health and Social Policy, King's College, London

Ruth Young, Fellow in Healthcare and Public Sector Management, Manchester Centre for Healthcare Management

Acknowledgements

The editors are grateful to the contributors to this collection and to Radcliffe Medical Press.

A note on terminology

In many of the following chapters, the terms 'service user' and 'carer' are used as generic terms to refer to people using social care services, NHS patients and those carers (family members, friends and neighbours) who care for them.

List of abbreviations

BCMHT	Black Country Mental Health Trust
CMHT	Community mental health team
CPA	Care programme approach
DHSS	Department of Health and Social Security
DoH	Department of Health
GMS	General medical services
GP	General practice/practitioner
HAZ	Health action zone
HMSO/TSO	Her Majesty's Stationery Office/The Stationery Office
HR	Human resources
HImP	Health improvement and modernisation plan
IM&T	Information management and technology
JCB	Joint Commissioning Board
LSP	Local strategic partnership
NatPact	National Primary and Care Trust Development Team
NHS	National Health Service
NSF	National service framework
OD	Organisational development
PCG/T	Primary care group/trust
PCP	Person-centred planning
PEC	Professional Executive Committee
PMS	Personal medical services
StHA	Strategic health authority
TUPE	Transfer of Undertakings (Protection of Employment) Regulations
VAT	Value added tax

Introduction

Jon Glasby and Edward Peck

In July 2000, the government's *NHS Plan* (DoH, 2000) set out a blueprint for the reform of English health services. Described by the Prime Minister and the Health Secretary as 'radical' and 'far reaching' (pp 9–16), *The NHS Plan* promised substantial extra investment in NHS facilities and staff and proposed significant changes in the organisation and delivery of healthcare. While most of the 144-page document focused on internal NHS issues, a four-page chapter on 'Changes between health and social services' examined the way in which the health service and local authorities were working together to provide co-ordinated services for people with both health and social care needs.

> If patients are to receive the best care, then the old divisions between health and social care need to be overcome. The NHS and social services do not always work effectively together as partners in care, so denying patients access to seamless services that are tailored to meet their particular needs. The division between health and social services can often be a source of confusion for people. Fundamental reforms are needed to tackle these problems.
>
> DoH, 2000, p 70

Amongst the reforms proposed was the concept of the care trust – a new level of primary care organisation that would commission and/or deliver both health and social care. Prior to this point, health and social services in the UK[1] had been organised separately, with the NHS responsible for healthcare and local authorities responsible for social care (*see* Box 1 for key differences between health and social care). As Glasby (2003, p 7) explains:

> In the UK, there are separate agencies responsible for meeting the health and social care needs of the population, with sharp and well documented divisions between the two types of organisation (*see*, for example, Glasby and Littlechild, 2000; Lewis, 2001). Although the definition of health and social care is contested and has changed over time, the British welfare state is based on the underlying assumption that it is possible to distinguish between people who are ill/injured (health needs) and people who need lower-level support due to frailty or disability (social needs). Whereas the former will be treated by the NHS, the latter will often fall under the remit of local authority [social

---

[1] With the exception of Northern Ireland, which has a more integrated health and social care structure.

services] departments. Under the current system, moreover, the former are likely to receive their care free of charge while the latter may be called upon to pay for the services they receive (and sometimes to pay considerable sums of money).

Now, for the first time, the government was proposing a new type of agency to bring both health and social care together into a single organisational entity, justifying its approach in terms of the need to 'remove the outdated institutional barriers between health and social services which have got in the way of people getting the care they need when they need it' (DoH, 2000, p 73). While many commentators have since discussed the various strengths and limitations of the policy being put forward, most people would agree that the proposal was an extremely significant one, with the potential to revolutionise the way in which public services are organised and provided.

Box 1 The health and social care divide

Social care
- Councillors democratically elected at a local level.
- Local government as a whole is overseen and monitored by the office of the Deputy Prime Minister (although the DoH has a significant role in the oversight and monitoring of social services departments).
- Subject to means-testing and charges.
- Based on specific geographical areas.
- Traditional focus on social factors contributing to individual situations and on choice/empowerment.
- Strong emphasis on social sciences.

NHS
- Non-executive directors appointed by central government.
- Overseen and monitored by DoH.
- Free at point of delivery.
- Boundaries are based on GP practice registration.
- Traditional emphasis on the individual and on medical cure.
- Strong emphasis on science.

Adapted from Glasby, 2003, p 10

Unfortunately, *The NHS Plan* was extremely short on detail. At this stage, care trusts were a completely untried model and were introduced in the document in four brief paragraphs (only 22 lines of text). From this, we could tell that care trusts were to be NHS bodies with the power to deliver social care services delegated from local authorities. They were also to be formed only where there was joint agreement that this model offered the best way to deliver services, although the government also signalled its intention to take powers to impose care trusts in areas which failed to work effectively in partnership. At the time it was envisaged that the first tranche of care trusts could be in place by 2001.

In addition to (and perhaps because of) this initial lack of detail, the care trust concept was also shrouded in controversy from the very beginning. Despite previous official policy documents ruling out structural reorganisation of health and social care (DoH, 1998), interventions by key players such as the NHS Confederation had raised the possibility of some form of integration and prompted considerable disagreement between health and social care agencies (such as the Local Government Association) as to whether the way forward lay in social care services being transferred to the NHS or in health services being transferred to local authorities.

Following *The NHS Plan*, further detail about the government's proposals was to emerge in a number of official documents (*see*, for example, DoH, 2001) and in the legislation designed to enact care trusts (the Health and Social Care Act 2001). Additional material has since appeared on the government's care trust website (www.doh.gov.uk/caretrusts/index.htm), providing guidance on issues such as estate and facilities management, human resources, financial issues and governance.

Essentially, care trusts are new NHS bodies, based either on primary care organisations or on NHS provider trusts, which are able to bring health and local government related services together into an integrated, single organisation (*see* Box 2 for

---

Box 2   Care trusts

'Care trusts are statutory NHS bodies, redesignated as care trusts under Section 45 of the Health and Social Care Act 2001. They build on PCTs [and] NHS trusts … They deliver integrated (whole systems) services in a single organisation. NHS and [local authority] health related functions are delegated to them, not transferred. They are able to commission and/or provide. They are voluntary – partners can withdraw.

Care trusts will be established on a voluntary basis and in partnership where there is a joint agreement at a local level that this model will offer the best way to deliver better health and social care services.

Service configuration will ensure the client group to be covered by the trust will be determined at a local level, although care trusts are likely to focus on specialist mental health and older people's services.

Care trusts will be able to commission, if they are a PCT based care trust, healthcare as well as local authority health related functions. They will also be able to deliver those services that the NHS organisation would normally provide, and local authority functions within the context of both models. Functions will be delivered under delegated authority from local authorities.

The introduction of care trusts is a real opportunity to deliver improved, integrated health and social care. It could see:

- An improvement in service provision and an integrated approach.
- A system which is designed around patient and users' needs.
- Better and clearer working arrangements for staff, with more and varied career opportunities.
- A single management structure, multi-disciplinary teams managed from one point, co-location of staff, as well as single or streamlined cross disciplinary assessments.
- Financial flexibility and efficiency from integration.
- A single strategic approach, with a single set of aims and targets.
- A stable organisational framework designed to improve quality of service provision through a single agency.'

DoH, 2002

further information). They are distinguished from traditional NHS trusts by having an extended board of up to 15 members in order to enable more local authority members and user and carer representatives to be formally involved in the governance of the organisation. Although guidance assumes that social care staff will transfer their employment to the NHS, some of the initial care trusts have opted to take these staff on secondment from the local authority (and in any event, as the Somerset Partnership Trust demonstrates in Chapter 3, other mechanisms exist for NHS trusts to employ social care staff).

Crucially, the power to compel care trusts has since been dropped by the government amid considerable opposition from the Local Government Association and front-line managers and practitioners, which found expression in the House of Lords, so the decision to form a care trust remains a voluntary one to be taken jointly by local health and social care agencies. In particular, much criticism of care trusts has come from social care providers and representatives fearful that a social care perspective will quickly become overshadowed by a much larger and more powerful health service based on a medical model of care (*see also* Chapters 6 and 7 for further detail on the nature, implementation and common criticisms of care trusts).

In the event, the formation of care trusts has proved slower than some in government may have expected and only four first-tranche care trusts were ready to 'go live' when the policy was formally introduced on 1 April 2002. These initial four have since been joined by a fifth care trust in October 2002 and by two more sites in April 2003 (*see* Box 3). With the exception of Northumberland and Braintree, the first care trusts were all focused on mental health services (an area where health and social care needs are often inextricably linked and where there is a relatively strong tradition of joint working between the NHS and social services). They were also based on previous provider mental health trusts in contrast to the primary care based models in Northumberland and Braintree.

Box 3   Early care trusts

April 2002 starters
- Bradford (mental health and learning disability services).
- Camden and Islington (mental health and learning disability services).
- Manchester (mental health services).
- Northumberland (commissioning all health and adult social care; providing primary and community and adult social care services [except working age mental health]).

October 2002 starters
- Witham, Braintree and Halstead (all local healthcare and health/social care for older people).

April 2003 starters
- Sandwell (mental health services).
- Sheffield (mental health and learning disability services).

At the time of writing an eighth care trust is proposed in Bexley, for older people and disabled people aged 18 and over.

Adapted from DoH care trust website

Ironically, *The NHS Plan* apparently envisaged an alternative organisational form for mental health providers bringing together health and social care provision – the combined mental health trust (DoH, 2000, p 122) – but this idea rapidly disappeared from view after its publication. In the event, most localities have pursued the creation of what are commonly known as 'partnership mental health NHS trusts' where the governance arrangements remain those of a traditional NHS trust, a director of social care is added to the board and staff seconded from the local authority (in part this secondment approach is determined by the Mental Health Act 1983 preventing so-called approved social workers being employed outside of the local authority).

Partnership working

Of course, the advent of care trusts is only one example of the current move towards much closer working between health and social care services. While the need for more effective inter-agency collaboration has long been recognised, the election of New Labour in May 1997 has signalled a much greater emphasis on partnerships as a guiding principle of public services. While we focus in much more detail on this issue in Chapter 1, it is important to recognise from the outset that the care trust model was developed and implemented against the background of a government committed to developing 'joined up solutions' to 'joined up problems'. Nor is this true only of health and social care – while this has been the subject of a number of policy initiatives, described in Chapter 1 of this book, there is also a much greater emphasis under New Labour on a range of wider partnerships, including:

- Partnerships between the public, private and voluntary sectors.
- Very broad partnerships that seek to address complex and engrained issues such as substance misuse, teenage pregnancy, regeneration, crime and disorder, and social exclusion.
- Partnerships between public services and the people who use these services (*see* Chapter 5).

For the purpose of this book, partnership is defined in terms of activity between health and social care agencies or practitioners where there is (Sullivan and Skelcher, 2002, pp 5–6):

- A shared responsibility for assessing the need for action, determining the type of action to be taken and agreeing the means of implementation.
- Negotiation between people from different agencies committed to working together over more than the short term.
- An intention to secure the delivery of benefits or added value which could not have been provided by a single agency acting alone.

The structure of this book

Against this background, we have sought to produce an edited collection of chapters designed to explore the care trust concept (and partnership working more generally) in more detail. To this end, the book is divided into two halves, with Part One focusing on our existing knowledge about partnership working between health and social care. In this section, Richard Poxton begins with an examination of the extensive literature on partnership working, summarising those factors that are thought to contribute to effective partnerships (Chapter 1). Next, Caroline Glendinning and colleagues summarise their findings from their evaluation of the Health Act 1999 (a piece of legislation designed to remove some of the legal and administrative barriers to partnership working and allow local agencies to work together more creatively and flexibly). In Chapter 3, Edward Peck and colleagues examine lessons from the creation of a health and social care trust within Somerset mental health services – a piece of inter-agency collaboration that was quoted as a good practice example in *The NHS Plan* (DoH, 2000). In Chapter 4, Nick Goodwin and Sue Peet explore the recent expansion of intermediate care services for older people, highlighting the similarities between this new way of working and the emerging care trust model. Finally, Chapter 5 provides a personal insight into the involvement of service users in health and social care partnerships from Diane Brodie, a mental health service user from Somerset, who was a board member of the Somerset Partnership Trust examined in Chapter 3. Comparing and contrasting her experiences with those of the researchers from the Somerset evaluation in Chapter 3 makes interesting and important reading, illustrating the diverse perspectives that different stakeholders bring to the partnership table and the potential for partnerships to have a negative as well as a positive impact. A service user perspective is also crucial in beginning to address a fundamental limitation in the existing partnership working literature: while much partnership working is justified in terms of better outcomes for users and carers, the views and experiences of users and carers are conspicuous by their absence from most of the partnership literature.

In Part Two, we turn attention specifically to care trusts, with a series of case studies and personal reactions to the care trust model. In Chapter 6, the DoH care trust lead, Shane Giles, offers a personal account of his work in supporting the creation of the first tranche of care trusts. For him, the care trust model is not about compulsion or about central control, but is simply an additional vehicle that local agencies need to consider and decide whether or not it is right for them. In contrast, Bob Hudson offers a detailed and robust critique of the care trust model in Chapter 7, arguing that the government's approach will not promote more effective partnership working and suggesting an alternative way forward. This is followed in Chapters 8 to 10 by a series of three case studies from different agencies in different areas of the country all trying to work more effectively across the health and social care boundary. This includes Northumberland (a first tranche care trust in April 2002), Sandwell (a health and social care community which formed a mental health care trust in April 2003, but which decided on a different route for learning disability services) and Hampshire (an area which considered care trust status and ruled it out in favour of other ways of working). Finally, Chapter 11 draws these various contributions together and identifies some overall themes and issues to inform our thinking about care trusts in the future. In particular, we feel that this book (and the wider partnership literature) raises some key questions and tensions which need further exploration. For example:

- Was the government correct to focus on developing new organisational structures to deliver its commitment to partnership working or should the emphasis have been on processes and relationships at a local level?

- Is there a danger of reorganisation fatigue with yet another structural change in health and social care?
- Is there a danger that social care perspectives will be lost in a much larger, more powerful and medically dominated NHS?
- Would it have been possible or desirable to compel care trust status on health and social care communities? Now that this power has been removed from legislation, is the government's intention still to take forward this notion of 'forced partnerships' and what will this mean for future policy and practice?
- What are the implications of the care trust model for relationships with the local authority, primary care and acute services?

Above all, however, the key issue is whether or not care trusts deliver improvements at ground level. Ultimately, our own view is that care trusts (and partnership working more generally) are a means to an end rather than an end in themselves – if a local care trust can demonstrate that it has led to improved services and outcomes for users and their carers, then it will have succeeded. If not, then the government's new model will have failed. At the time of writing (mid-2003), the jury is still out.

References

Department of Health (1998) *Partnership in Action: new opportunities for joint working between health and social services – a discussion document.* Department of Health, London.

Department of Health (2000) *The NHS Plan: a plan for investment, a plan for reform.* TSO, London.

Department of Health (2001) *Care Trusts: emerging framework.* DoH, London.

Department of Health (2002) *Care Trusts: background briefing.* Available online via www.doh.gov.uk/caretrusts/infobackground.htm (accessed 09/04/03).

Glasby J (2003) *Hospital Discharge: integrating health and social care.* Radcliffe Medical Press, Oxford.

Glasby J and Littlechild R (2000) *The Health and Social Care Divide: the experiences of older people.* PEPAR Publications, Birmingham.

Lewis J (2001) Older people and the health-social care boundary in the UK: half a century of hidden policy conflict. *Social Policy and Administration.* **35**(4): 343–59.

Sullivan H and Skelcher C (2002) *Working Across Boundaries: collaboration in public services.* Palgrave, Basingstoke.

PART ONE

Partnership working

The first half of this book explores our existing knowledge about partnership working, much of which will apply to health and social care communities wishing to establish, or at least consider, care trusts. For example, those agencies that have been working together to develop intermediate care services, to pool financial resources or to integrate provision will all have encountered barriers and learned lessons that may equally apply to care trusts.

In particular, Part One covers:

- existing lessons from the partnership working literature (Chapter 1)
- the national evaluation of the Health Act flexibilities (Chapter 2)
- the evaluation of the Somerset Mental Health Partnership Trust (Chapter 3)
- the national evaluation of intermediate care (Chapter 4)
- a service user perspective on user involvement in health and social care partnerships (Chapter 5).

What makes effective partnerships between health and social care?

Richard Poxton

The New Labour government which came to power in 1997 was determined to address the failure of public agencies to work together and espoused a political philosophy based more on collaboration than on competition. Frank Dobson (the then Secretary of State) famously stated his intent to break down the 'Berlin Wall' between the NHS and social services. This determination was crucially within the wider policy agenda of social inclusion that places health and social care as supporting partners in a wider mission. Thus, the Public Health Green Paper (DoH, 1998a) outlined the role of the NHS not just in terms of 'curing' and treating the ill, but rather as part of a network of public functions concerned with promoting a full and healthy lifestyle – alongside local government, employment agencies and others.

The specific policy framework applying to health and social care subsequently built in proposals to operationalise this intent. The NHS and social services (DoH, 1998b, 1999a) White Papers proposed placing a 'duty of partnership' on each agency, while health authorities and PCGs were required to have representation on their boards from the local authority. More flexible ways of working across agencies were introduced in the *Partnership in Action* discussion document (DoH, 1998c; *see also* Chapter 2). As an example of the current emphasis on partnership working, a series of New Labour policy initiatives are set out in Box 1.1.

Box 1.1 Partnership working under New Labour

Partnership initiatives include:

- A duty of partnership between health and social care.
- Joint planning frameworks (such as joint investment plans between health and local government with regard to continuing and community care services, or health improvement and modernisation plans (HImPs) for improving local health and healthcare).

- New powers to enable health and social care agencies to work together more flexibly (for example, by pooling budgets or integrating provision; *see* Chapter 2 for further discussion).
- New intermediate care services to prevent unnecessary hospital admissions, facilitate swift hospital discharges and prevent premature admission to long-term residential or nursing care (*see* Chapter 4).
- Single assessments for older people so that they do not have to give the same personal information to a large number of different health and social care professionals during assessments.
- Integrated community equipment stores.
- Health action zones (HAZs) to improve the health of local communities in areas of high social exclusion.
- New national service frameworks (NSFs) applicable to both health and social services to ensure consistent access to services and quality of care across the country. The first frameworks focus on mental health, coronary heart disease and services for older people.
- Overarching strategic frameworks (local strategic partnerships (LSPs)) to bring together key players locally from the public, private and voluntary sectors (*see later* in this chapter).
- New children's trusts to integrate health, education and social care (*see* Chapter 11 for further discussion).

As a result of New Labour's emphasis on partnership working, an array of new joint working has begun to develop at an operational level, including joint investment plans, joint assessments of older people's needs and the establishment of joint rehabilitation schemes. However, the question remains as to whether the policies described in Box 1.1 will be sufficient by themselves to overcome the obstacles that have prevented previous efforts such as joint commissioning from having a greater impact. Also, this emphasis on partnership working between health and social care came at a time when local NHS agencies (increasingly with PCTs at the fore) and social services departments were increasingly being required to work more closely with other areas of local government, as well as with other public agencies and independent and voluntary organisations. Health and social care had struggled with different aspects of partnership working for several decades. The new challenge was not only to make quick and sustainable progress here, but also to make new alliances that would contribute to broader aspects of community and individual well-being.

The purpose of partnerships

One problem in any consideration of what makes for effective partnerships is trying to address the issue of their purpose. If it is clear what partnerships are trying to achieve then it should be less difficult (at least) to determine the degree of success. This challenge is compounded when there is less than total clarity over what is meant by partnership in the first place.

According to one evaluation of a partnership working initiative (Glendinning *et al.*, 2002; *see also* Chapter 2), partnerships are often established in order to:

- improve efficiency (reduce duplication, use scarce resources better)
- provide more flexible, seamless patterns of services
- redistribute services more equitably across the locality
- enhance the experiences of service users.

Additionally the Audit Commission (1998) has emphasised the importance of partnerships in addressing 'wicked issues' such as avoidable hospital admission for older people, as well as the inherent benefit of better co-ordinated services and less organisational fragmentation. More recently the partnership guidance for the learning disability White Paper *Valuing People* (DoH, 2001) has drawn attention to the impact of services on the lives of individuals. The purpose of partnership here is to achieve social inclusion for people with learning disabilities, based upon enabling them to lead fulfilling lives. This fundamental approach to partnership contains three key elements:

- the aspects of people's lives embraced by partnership arrangements must encompass all aspects of a person's aspirations (not just health and social care)
- the organisations involved in the partnership must therefore include all those with an interest or responsibility across this full range of issues (at strategic as well as operational management and practitioner levels)
- the partnership must operate with the person with a learning disability and their wishes and interests at the centre of the decision-making process.

In other policy areas both the extent and the specific applications of partnership working is now much clearer. For example, the *National Service Framework for Mental Health* (DoH, 1999b) made specific requirements in respect of integrated working at practitioner team level. It has also provided a major impetus for the development not just of partnership working between professionals, but also for the design of integrated systems that seek to present a 'one stop' approach to users. Local mental health NSF implementation teams have been set up involving the acute in-patient, community and primary care components of the local NHS together with social services, users, carers and local voluntary agencies. One of the performance measures against which these implementation teams have been assessed and rated by the DoH is the extent to which formal partnership arrangements (e.g. joint management) have been put in place; an early example of partnership working slipping from the permissive category into the obligatory one (*see* Chapter 11 for further discussion of this phenomenon).

It is also clear from more recent guidance that partnership should be broadened to include education providers, the Employment Agency, Income Support, the Learning and Skills Council, housing associations and others that have a part to play in meeting the comprehensive needs of users. The NSF was also established on the basis of a clear set of values that includes the need to increase the participation of users in the planning and delivery of care (*see* Chapter 5).

The NHS Plan remains one of the most important policy frameworks within which partnership working is required to operate (DoH, 2000). It offers the prospect of integration within significant parts of the health and social care systems. The emphasis is on the integration of services, whilst also leaving the door open for organisational reconfiguration. However, *The NHS Plan* has been criticised as focusing too much on hospital provision within the NHS and not doing enough to promote the notion of real 'whole systems' working that properly embraces community and primary care services as well as acute: there is still more than a hint of getting hospitals to work more efficiently and all will be well.

But for older people's services in particular *The NHS Plan* gives some important directives on what partnership working should cover, including the following:

- a continuing development of a range of intermediate care services designed to cut down the time that people have to spend in hospital (*see* Chapter 4)
- exploring ways of reducing both the costs and the institutionalised approach to long-term care
- more emphasis on the promotion of healthy ageing and reducing the impact of disabilities
- placing the notion of rehabilitation at the heart of older people's health and social care services: enabling older people to function at their optimal level regardless of their age or other circumstances
- ensuring that an engagement with users and carers drives policy, practice and service developments (*see* Chapter 5)
- service reforms that should include: joint health and social care assessments, personal care plans for certain groups of older people, integrated teams working from the same location and 'one stop shop' points of entry to the system.

Partnership working in practice

These policy frameworks (with partnership at the core) place the onus for determining ways forward upon local partners, but generally within a tightly defined set of expectations and process requirements. A common theme is that of organisations performing as though they were an integrated whole, even though they remain organisationally separate:

- at a strategic level, agencies are required to plan together and share information about the use of resources, for example through HImPs and joint investment plans
- at the level of operational management, a range of policies require a demonstration of partnership, for example, the Mental Health NSF expects integrated specialist health and social care teams, and the Older People's NSF requires the implementation of a single assessment process that covers health and social care needs
- at the level of individual care and support, these operational requirements are taken further with expectations of a single point of access, shared information systems and joint training across health and social care staff.

Managing across professional and agency boundaries is a fundamental issue in the drive for 'joined up' health and social care. But real achievements will be made only if there is clarity around goals and outcomes for users of services, and if managing across boundaries is part of a broader approach that works at all levels of organisational decision making. For reasons of both effectiveness and efficiency there has been increasing attention given to breaking down old ways of working and replacing these with processes and practices that have users' needs at the core.

In many ways the services that faced the government when it came to power in 1997 (despite the skills and commitment of many practitioners and managers) could be typified as having:

- multiple entry points
- unwieldy assessments
- user unfriendly care management
- too much emphasis on dependency
- unnecessary admissions to and delayed discharges from hospital
- funding disputes.

Whilst the health and social care system had:

- duplication of effort
- inconsistent collaboration
- limited finance and skills
- lack of community-based and out-of-hours services
- incoherent access arrangements
- confusing lines of responsibility.

The challenge to managers was how to respond positively to these challenges so that enthusiastic staff were further encouraged whilst reluctant ones were supported in new ways of working. To be able to do this effectively, managers must be aware both of the big picture – the national and local strategic agenda – and the practicalities of joint working on the ground.

In addition, the government has introduced LSPs to bring together under one umbrella the different parts of the public sector and the private, business, voluntary and community sectors. Key tasks include the need to operate at a level that enables strategic decisions to be taken, whilst still being close enough to individual neighbourhoods to allow action to be determined at community level, and the need to create strengthened, empowered and safer communities. LSPs are non-statutory, non-executive organisations – they are intended to be powerful, but through their influence and their networking rather than any executive powers in law. At the time of writing (mid-2003), the implications for relationships between local authorities and the local NHS are still far from clear. However, LSPs are potentially very significant for partnership working and assign key roles to local NHS agencies. These include:

- aligning different health and local government planning mechanisms
- ensuring properly co-ordinated NHS input
- determining with other members of the health community how health interests should be represented on the LSP
- developing local strategies for national and local priorities.

Increasingly the push for bigger and better partnerships recognises that people's needs do not fit neatly within one agency's responsibilities. There is increasing recognition that an integrated or whole systems approach is required, with services organised around users. This would also involve all participants accepting their interdependence and that actions in one part of the system have an inevitable impact elsewhere.

Within this context, partnerships become important both across and within agencies. A consequence of this is that it is the collaborative effort that is important rather than the organisational design. As a result there is growing emphasis on partnership working which concentrates on users' pathways or journeys through the various care systems – enabling older people to continue living in their own homes, ensuring that any stay in hospital is only for as long as necessary, helping them to recover and maintain an optimal level of capability. In organisational terms there is a spectrum of connections between agencies:

- **communication**: informing each other of separate actions
- **co-ordination**: working separately, but mindful of each other's actions
- **collaboration**: working together in a cohesive way
- **integration**: working together as one agency.

Overall, the key message is that partnerships are intended to respond to a wide range of cross-cutting and complex social problems such as unemployment, poverty and poor health. As a result, organisational responses have to be similarly subtle, complex and inter-connected if they are to be effective. Indeed, a socially inclusive vision of people's lives (e.g. as outlined in *Valuing People*) means that there will always be a complex web of organisations and individuals that need to work together in the interests of service users and carers. It is not feasible to turn that complexity into a simple, linear arrangement in either organisational or process terms. As a result, ways forward are likely to be complex rather than 'neat'.

Key ingredients

Given the fluid state of partnerships described above, it is unsurprising that evidence on what makes for success is rather thin on the ground. Nevertheless, on the basis of various studies, it is possible to gain a view of what helps and what hinders.

What helps

Partnerships between agencies have to face up to an array of differences: political structures, accountability systems, ways of considering the needs of patients and users, statutory responsibilities, professional backgrounds of those charged with making it work, and the different operations, customs and practices that permeate working arrangements (e.g. regarding confidentiality, case closure, file destruction, complaints, etc.).

Structures are required that translate needs-based information into changes that impact on service design and delivery. This requires inter-agency ownership of decisions to commit resources to meet the wide range of needs of individual users and their carers. Without this connection between policy makers and practitioners, effective, jointly managed and operated multi-disciplinary teams are unlikely to be viable. Clarity about respective areas of responsibility and lines of accountability is required from the outset.

But successful partnerships require more than the 'right' structural design. Research and experience highlights the key partnership challenges as being around culture and organisational behaviour, not around structures (Hudson and Hardy, 2002; Peck *et al.*, 2001). It is comparatively easy to develop and establish joint structures, policies and protocols. The real issue is that of whether individuals and organisations can work in new ways that mean partnerships are genuine and sustainable. Attempts by agencies to create inter-agency structures without paying attention to the 'building blocks' of partnership will almost certainly lead to those arrangements falling down when early difficulties arise. Essentially we are dealing with complex organisational systems and practitioner/clinician change.

These building blocks have been described by Greig and Poxton (2001) in terms of a 'Partnership Readiness Framework' (*see* Box 1.2). This identifies a series of factors that underpin effective partnerships and can be used by front-line agencies to consider their current readiness for partnership working and what they may need to do in order to get beyond the planning stage and survive early difficulties. In similar vein, the Nuffield Institute for Health has developed a partnership asessment tool (Hardy *et al.*, 2000) based upon extensive empirical research that can be used as a local working tool.

Box 1.2   The Partnership Readiness Framework

- Building shared values and principles.
- Agreeing specific policy shifts.
- Being prepared to explore new service options.
- Determining agreed boundaries.
- Agreeing respective roles with regard to commissioning, purchasing and providing.
- Identifying agreed resource pools.
- Ensuring effective leadership.
- Providing sufficient development capacity.
- Developing and sustaining good personal relationships.
- Paying specific attention to mutual trust and attitude.

Greig and Poxton, 2001

A further important lesson from past studies is the need to recognise the multi-layered nature of partnership working when it is put into action. Decisions are taken at various levels within and outside organisations. Gaining better outcomes for individuals and communities depends on these levels working together in a reasonably cohesive way. It is crucial to be able to pinpoint those key layers of decision-making and the essential infrastructure that underpins them (*see* Box 1.3). Most crucially, attention must be paid to the linkages between these different elements, so that effective inter-agency work at one level is not undermined by its failure to be translated into joint action at another. Understanding decision-making processes is a fundamental ingredient of effective working within and between agencies.

Box 1.3 Ensuring effective partnerships

- The establishment of **strategic partnerships** that set the overarching framework and objectives for the services in question and that meet the necessary governance requirements.
- Means of **engaging with users and other local people**, including those beyond traditional service boundaries, in ways that make sense to them and that are properly impacting on key resource and other decision making.
- Ways of **promoting ownership** of the partnership from leaders, managers and staff through effective communication and a sharing of the potential benefits.
- Clarity over how significant shifts in service patterns are to be achieved through the **planning and operationalisation** of key strategic decisions that require macro changes in service design.
- Inter-agency **assessment systems** that ensure shared ownership of decisions to commit resources to meet the holistic needs of individuals.
- Networks or systems that facilitate integrated **information and other supports** at an individual and aggregate level.
- The **sharing of resources** through pooled budgets and other means.
- A comprehensive **shared local training** policy and programmes.
- Joint **workforce planning** mechanisms that consider how to develop a workforce that can both deliver and strategically commission services.
- An **integrated monitoring and review system** that results in a shared understanding of the effectiveness of current services, and thus the evidence base for changes in the future.
- A clear and shared **performance and audit** approach to provide publicly visible shared ownership of decisions and the use of resources.

In addition, managers and others charged with the implementation of partnership working have to learn how to work *with* inherent and unavoidable organisational complexity, rather than trying to remove it in ways that will make delivering on that complexity impossible. A greater understanding and then nurturing of the effective levers for change are crucial aspects of the way forward. Similarly, many partnership arrangements are still embarked upon more from a desire to establish joint working per se, than a clear understanding of how they might improve people's lives. Unless partners are clear from an early stage about what aspects of services and people's lives the new arrangements are designed to improve, any structural changes are likely to achieve little real change.

What hinders

Experience of partnership working has shown that progress can be helped or hindered by a combination of contextual factors. Each place has its own unique selection of issues, or positions, on the same issues. Having examined some factors that assist partnership implementation, it is also important to be clear about those that can get in the way. These are summarised in Box 1.4 from research

---

Box 1.4   Barriers to effective partnership working

- Structural (the fragmentation of service responsibilities across and within agency boundaries).
- Procedural (differences in planning and budget cycles).
- Financial (differences in funding mechanisms and resource flows).
- Professional (differences in ideologies, values and professional interests).
- Perceived threats to status, autonomy and legitimacy.

Hardy *et al.*, 1992

---

conducted during the 1990s at the Nuffield Institute of Health, University of Leeds.

In addition, there is a growing agenda, not just for 'joined up' working, but for a structural integration of organisations (and of the various teams of practitioners within them). However, the little evidence that exists from the Northern Ireland experience of health and social care organisational integration suggests that this solves little by itself and still requires significant emphasis on joint working between different component parts (DoH, Social Services and Public Safety, 2000). The real risk is that organisations will opt for some form of reconfiguration that satisfies government requirements but falls short of the real change needed for true partnership. Whilst it is reasonably clear that stable long-term and trusting relationships are crucial for sustainable joined up working, the pressures are all for quick results and specific targets. In some cases, there may be an argument for less ambitious partnerships based more upon mutual self-interest than longer-term vision. What matters is what works and this means being clear about the better outcomes that are being sought for local communities and for individual users and patients. Partnerships are likely to continue to come in many forms – there really are no neat and tidy solutions. What is important is to recognise what particular ways forward may be appropriate, based upon a keen awareness of the local circumstances.

But whilst the government has gone some way to removing many of the structural barriers to developing partnerships, a host of other cultural and professional barriers remain. Conceptual differences between professionals are often cited as barriers in relation to the provision of care, for example in differences of opinion concerning the medical versus social model in the area of mental health or in different conceptual understandings of rehabilitation for older people. Communication problems are also often cited in inquiries as one of the contributing factors to the breakdown of care; this can be due to lack of mutual understanding of professionals' roles. However, reaching a shared understanding of concepts amongst people from different organisational and professional backgrounds is unlikely to be achieved by merely adopting a particular process.

Moving ahead

To date, many places have adopted cross-agency decision-making and management arrangements to promote and facilitate partnership working. These structural aspects are necessary in order to formalise the sharing of decision-making powers between otherwise separately accountable organisations and their respective staff. But it is important to stress that there is no right answer in terms of what structure to adopt – different solutions will suit different places. Finding a structure or model to support local services or integrated team development does not of itself ensure better outcomes for service users. Nor does it necessarily ensure better partnership working.

So how can the 'right' approach to a partnership model be adopted? Essentially what is 'right' is what works – i.e. the framework that effectively brings together decision makers at strategic, operational management and practitioner levels in a coherent needs-focused manner to ensure the most effective deployment of resources (of all kinds). Of course other aspects are important, not least how practitioners organise their time and skills with service users and how they relate to colleagues in other agencies. Overall, it may be possible to get a sense of the 'right' approach by considering the following issues.

- **What achievements are being sought?** A large, ambitious agenda for change, covering a number of care groups, is likely to benefit from a significant piece of partnership decision-making machinery that includes a strategic level component, probably involving councillors and non-executive directors. A smaller scale programme that is focused on individual services or a project approach will not require such sophistication and could operate at a lower level of delegated powers.
- **What is the local history of partnership working?** It is important to be mindful of previous successes and setbacks in establishing similar ways of working, so as to build upon existing strengths and also to mainstream informal arrangements. In doing this building up, it is important not to aim too high too quickly – having a structure that is sustainable is crucial; reluctant participants can jeopardise progress and such issues should be addressed before ploughing ahead with an ambitious structure.
- **What does the current organisational and political geography tell you?** It is important to be able to identify and build upon 'natural' decision-making focal points that already work, whether these be localities within a wider geographical area or a particular grouping of like-minded agencies or individuals. Provider organisations should be respected and afforded a prominent position in the local arrangements that reflects their willingness to act in a non-competitive manner.
- **How does organisational reconfiguration affect partnership structures?** Partnership development is significantly about creating systems and ways of working that will survive and thrive regardless of the organisational and personnel changes that will inevitably continue to go on around them. But the continuing process of change does demand time and effort from senior and other staff, and it is important to be realistic about this when designing new partnership arrangements.
- **How important is the current strength of local partnerships?** As often stated, but too rarely observed, form should follow function. By undertaking an honest audit of the strength of local partnership working (e.g. by a shared 'scoring' of the various components of the Partnership Readiness Framework) it should be possible to design a model that reflects both current circumstances and future

aspirations; the degree of shared (effectively integrated) decision-making, especially involving resources, should grow as partnership strength develops.

- **How broad should the local partnership structure be?** All of the above points continue to apply, but it is clear that partnership has to involve more than the NHS and social services; local structures and models should allow for this outward-looking element, involving other local authority departments and other parts of the public services. Inevitably to do this in a meaningful way it will be important to ensure that the success of the model is not dependent simply on what happens at meetings. Partnership working is more about what happens between meetings than the 'signing off' that takes place at them.

- **How should users, carers, the independent sector and local communities be involved in the partnership model?** The strength of a local partnership can be said to be determined by the extent of real power sharing that takes place. In practice this is constrained to an extent by the fact that the statutory commissioning and purchasing agencies can delegate their powers only to each other but do not lose their accountability. Local non-statutory partners can, of course, bring a great deal to the partnership arrangement, in terms of needs assessment and determining appropriate responses, and local models and structures should facilitate this involvement rather than deter it. As always, rather than the nature of the model it will be the depth of the commitment to working together and sharing decision making that determines whether their involvement is successful or not.

References

Audit Commission (1998) *A Fruitful Partnership: effective partnership working*. Audit Commission, London.

Department of Health (1998a) *Our Healthier Nation: a contract for health*. TSO, London.

Department of Health (1998b) *The New NHS: modern, dependable*. TSO, London.

Department of Health (1998c) *Partnership in Action: new opportunities for joint working between health and social services – a discussion document*. DoH, London.

Department of Health (1999a) *Modernising Social Services: promoting independence, improving protection, raising standards*. TSO, London.

Department of Health (1999b) *National Service Framework for Mental Health*. DoH, London.

Department of Health (2000) *The NHS Plan: a plan for investment, a plan for reform*. TSO, London.

Department of Health (2001) *Valuing People: a new strategy for learning disability for the 21st century*. TSO, London.

Department of Health, Social Services and Public Safety (2000) *Facing the Future: building on the lessons of winter 1999/2000*. Department of Health, Social Services and Public Safety, Belfast.

Glendinning C, Hudson B, Hardy B *et al.* (2002) *National Evaluation of Notifications for Use of the Section 31 Partnership Flexibilities of the Health Act 1999: final project report*.

National Primary Care Research and Development Centre and Nuffield Institute for Health, Manchester/Leeds.

Greig R and Poxton R (2001) From joint commissioning to partnership working – will the new policy framework make a difference? *Managing Community Care.* **9**(4): 32–8.

Hardy B, Hudson B and Waddington E (2000) *What Makes a Good Partnership? A Partnership Assessment Tool.* Nuffield Institute for Health/NHS Executive Trent Region, Leeds.

Hardy B, Turrell A and Wistow G (1992) *Innovations in Community Care Management.* Avebury, Aldershot.

Hudson B and Hardy B (2002) What is a 'successful' partnership and how can it be measured? In: C Glendinning, M Powell and K Rummery (eds) *Partnerships, New Labour and the Governance of Welfare.* Policy Press, Bristol.

Peck E, Towell D and Gulliver P (2001) The meanings of culture in health and social care: a study of the combined trust in Somerset. *J Interprofessional Care.* **15**(4): 319–27.

CHAPTER 2

The Health Act 1999 section 31 partnership 'flexibilities'

Caroline Glendinning, Bob Hudson,
Brian Hardy and Ruth Young

Introduction: background to the Health Act 1999

The 'flexibilities' contained in section 31 of the Health Act 1999 remove some of the formal barriers that have long been alleged to impede closer collaboration between the NHS and local authority services. They also provide the essential legal mechanism for constructing the constitutional framework of care trusts. The experiences of the first sites to use these new flexibilities therefore offer valuable insights into the problems and benefits that are also likely to characterise care trusts.

The problematic relationships between NHS and local authority services have been alleged (Lewis, 2001; Means *et al.*, 2002) to originate in the welfare state structures of the late 1940s, in which hospital and GP services formed part of the newly created NHS while community health services were the responsibility of local authorities. A major reorganisation in 1974 transferred the latter to the NHS but, although this may have improved the integration of health services, it nevertheless sharpened the boundaries between these and the remaining local authority social and welfare services (Hudson and Henwood, 2002). Subsequent attempts to improve collaboration across the NHS–local authority boundary through joint finance and joint planning mechanisms were stimulated by pressures from the early 1980s onwards to move people with learning disabilities and mental illness from long-stay hospitals to the community. Although some successes were reported in relation to small scale and marginal activities, any impact on the mainstream activities of either health or social services organisations was rare (Audit Commission, 1986; Nocon, 1994). Meanwhile, the major inflow of social security resources into the supply of private residential and nursing home facilities for older people during the decade up to 1993 provided little incentive for collaboration, as both the NHS and local authorities 'could now simply be bypassed' (Hudson and Henwood, 2002, p 156).

The 1993 community care reforms were intended to reduce fragmentation and the diffusion of responsibilities for community care services by unequivocally assigning lead responsibility to local authority social services. However, again it is arguable that this consolidation *within* local authority social services took place at the expense of collaboration *between* social services and health. Moreover, the simultaneous introduction of quasi-markets within both sectors greatly increased the challenges of co-ordination by introducing competition between providers (Wistow and Hardy, 1996) and contracts that specified provider responsibilities and thus sharpened service boundaries (Glendinning, 1998). Furthermore, major elements of both health and social care – GP services, many acute and hospital services, and virtually all other local authority services – remained outside of virtually all collaborative initiatives.

With the New Labour government that came to power in May 1997, partnership and collaboration quickly became mantras within political and policy discourses. Partnerships – between organisations, sectors, services and even between purchasers and providers – were promoted as the alternative to the adversarial relationships of the former quasi-market (Clarke and Glendinning, 2002). Implicit in this shift was the assumption that partnership would be a more effective mechanism than the contracts of the former quasi-market for improving co-ordination between services. Moreover, collaboration was no longer a marginal option, but 'was at the very heart of new policies on health and social care' (Hudson and Henwood, 2002, p 157).

Partnerships, *Partnership in Action* and the Health Act

The New Labour government's proposals to tackle the barriers to closer collaboration between the NHS and social care services first appeared in a discussion document, *Partnership in Action* (DoH, 1998). This highlighted the need for closer joint working at the different levels of strategic planning, service commissioning and front-line service provision. It proposed three new 'flexibilities' – relaxations of the normal statutory boundaries and responsibilities – that were subsequently incorporated into section 31 of the Health Act 1999:

- **pooled budgets:** Resources contributed to the pool by the partner organisations would lose their distinctive health or social service identity; health or social services staff could decide how pooled resources were spent across the spectrum of health or social care services
- **lead commissioning:** Here one partner would delegate its commissioning responsibilities (and associated resources) to the other partner, who would then commission an integrated range of health and social care services on behalf of both
- **integrated provision:** This would allow a single statutory organisation to provide both health and social care services and employ the appropriate range of staff to do so

Although *Partnership in Action* focused on the NHS–social services boundary, the subsequent legislation was extended to other local authority services such as education and housing, as long as these had some health-related function. On the NHS side, statutory partners could include (until April 2002) health authorities,

PCTs and NHS trusts. However, guidance accompanying the legislation stressed that other organisations (such as the police and probation services and independent sector providers) could – indeed should – be involved, although they could not legally hold a pooled budget or act as lead commissioners.

The section 31 flexibilities, together with two other sections of the 1999 Health Act that also freed up restrictions on the transfer of resources between NHS and local authority sectors (Hudson and Henwood, 2002), provide the legal underpinnings for care trusts. It is for this reason that the lessons learnt from the implementation of the Health Act flexibilities are so important in this book.

Implementing the Health Act flexibilities

The flexibilities could be used from April 2000. Prospective partnerships are required to register their intended use of the flexibilities with their NHS regional office (strategic health authority (StHA) since April 2002). Registrations are forwarded to the Joint Health and Social Care Unit at the DoH and subsequently published on its website. Initially, it was anticipated that up to 100 sites would use the flexibilities from the earliest opportunity in April 2000. In fact, notifications to the DoH were much slower, and by November 2000 only 32 had been received. Moreover, six of these were for short-term 'winter pressures' initiatives and a further two were only general expressions of interest, not firm intentions. However, new partnerships have continued to develop and, by January 2003, 187 had been notified to the DoH. Although use of the flexibilities (and the choice of combinations – one, two or all three, simultaneously or in succession) remains optional, the Health Act 1999 gives the Secretary of State for Health powers to mandate their use in certain circumstances.

The DoH commissioned an evaluation of the Health Act flexibilities, based on the first 32 notifications (Glendinning *et al.*, 2002). The evaluation included:

- a baseline postal survey of all notifications, with a follow-up survey 18 months later
- Case studies of 10 partnerships, selected to cover the widest range of services, budget size, organisational complexity and combination of the flexibilities themselves
- follow-up in-depth case studies of three of these sites, where the implications of using the flexibilities appeared most far-reaching.[1]

The baseline postal survey of the first notifications revealed that the most common combination of partners was a health authority, NHS trust and local authority social services department. Pooled budgets were the most popular flexibility, either singly or in combination with another flexibility. The flexibilities were most often being used to integrate services for people with learning disabilities (reflecting the long history of joint working for this group), older people (particularly new intermediate care and 'rapid response' services) and mental health services. Very few partnerships involved services for children (mainly child and adolescent

---

[1] Three interim reports of the evaluation (Hudson *et al.*, 2001, 2002a,b) contain full details of the samples and sites, and the survey and case study findings.

mental health services), drug and alcohol misuse services, services for adults and/or children with physical or sensory impairments or community equipment services. The same patterns of flexibilities, partner organisations and services were evident in a subsequent analysis of all the notifications received by the DoH by April 2002, two years after implementation (Glendinning *et al.*, 2002).

The first sites notifying their use of the flexibilities were followed up with a second postal survey after 18 months. This revealed some substantial developments: partnerships were broadening to include new PCT partners and some new services and user groups were being drawn in. Although many achievements were focused on overcoming difficulties in the processes of establishing the partnership, some outcome-oriented achievements were cited, including the establishment of new organisational and commissioning arrangements, new staff appointments and greater involvement of users and carers. Plans to further extend the use of the flexibilities to include other services and users were also widespread.

However, the follow-up survey also hinted at some of the challenges in implementing the flexibilities, particularly in relation to the sharing of information between partners (including problems with the quality and compatibility of data and IT systems), continuing cultural and other differences between partner organisations and resource shortages by one or more partners. It was also clear that progress on the full implementation of the integrated provider flexibility (including integrating management and operational systems and transferring employment) was slower than the other two flexibilities. The case studies revealed some of the reasons for these difficulties.

Origins of the partnership and the decision to use the flexibilities

Most partnerships had built on long local histories of collaboration; the flexibilities therefore offered the opportunity to progress well-established local collaborative strategies. Only a minority of partnerships had deliberately used the notification process to 'kick start' problematic local inter-sectoral relationships. These different histories impacted on the subsequent pace of change; partnerships with less well-grounded collaborative histories had to work particularly hard to build up trust, especially in financial matters.

Factors which helped the decision to use the flexibilities included:

- high and broadly equal levels of commitment to the partnership among the main partner organisations
- perceived equity in the financial situations of the partner organisations
- co-terminous geographical boundaries between local health and social services organisations
- senior managers with clear vision and commitment to the partnership
- 'dense' and stable local networks in which key individuals had built up shared working histories and continued to interact in many different contexts
- senior and/or middle managers with time and skills to commit to the partnership
- health action zones, which provided experience of collaborative working, facilitation and sometimes financial support as well

- the transition by local PCGs to trust status, which could be an opportunity for wider reorganisation around a section 31 partnership.

Significantly, prospective partnerships did not need to be well-resourced; indeed, some saw it as an opportunity to make more efficient use of the very scarce resources of all partners.

> I knew for a fact that there were hugely defensive modes of operation going on … and it struck us that if we could have all that money in one pot, all of that [disagreement] in theory should disappear and we should also be able to, in a more sensible way, manage that resource and produce quicker results in terms of provision.

However (perceived) equality in partners' financial situations was important.

> [This area] is relatively poorly resourced on both sides – and therefore coming together as a partnership was less problematic on the basis of if you haven't got a rich partner then you don't need some kind of prenuptial agreement. You actually came together as joint partners that were stretched for resources.

The challenges of implementing the Health Act flexibilities

Legal arrangements

Section 31 partnerships had to be underpinned by appropriate legal frameworks that could safeguard the probity of the partnership as well as the partner organisations' own statutory responsibilities. Partnerships that were based on established, good, informal relationships initially saw these legal frameworks as unnecessarily heavy-handed, formal and a threat to the culture of collaboration. Local authority legal and finance staff, in particular, could be unpopular for their insistence on tight accountability, probity and risk management frameworks.

However, with hindsight, respondents appreciated the importance of clear legal and financial frameworks, particularly when setting up pooled budgets and integrated provider organisations which were described as 'really scary' and 'hugely complex'. Clear legal frameworks were also important in contexts of organisational complexity, where opportunities for organisational learning were restricted. For example, in one county the section 31 legal framework and manual developed by the social services department and health authority provided a template for other partnerships in the area that brought in district councils and PCTs. However, the development of legal and financial frameworks was an ongoing process that had to respond to wider organisational changes; the abolition of health authorities and the rapid move from PCG to PCT status had meant some major adjustments for some partnerships. As well as establishing formal arrangements for the horizontal relationships between NHS and local authority partners, agreement also had to be reached about the new relationships and responsibilities of the commissioning and provider elements of the partnership, with matters such as budget monitoring, information sharing and user charges incorporated into contracts or service level agreements.

Financial arrangements

Although the most widely used of the section 31 flexibilities, managing pooled budgets also presented major challenges. Some sites reported difficulties in determining the size of the partners' respective contributions; historic budgets could not simply be transferred if these included regular overspends or deficits, without threats to trust.

> Would you get married to someone knowing they had a huge overdraft?

Differences in NHS and local government financial management systems had to be overcome; local government financial accountability systems were generally much tighter, making it easier to identify costs and expenditure patterns. However, this also led to cultural differences that were reinforced by the attitudes of local authority councillors and front-line staff.

> I think there are different cultures between the way health and social services look at financial controls; budgetary control is foremost in the minds of social services and council staff; it isn't necessarily the case in health services.

The different timing of financial planning and audit arrangements (December for local government, August for NHS organisations) – described as '180 degrees different' – was a major problem in planning pooled budgets. Partnerships also had to reconcile the different value added tax (VAT) regimes in local authorities and the NHS, as the choice of lead agency for VAT purposes had significant financial consequences. However, these problems were largely resolved by the publication of guidance from the DoH and Customs and Excise.

As pooled budgets bedded down, new challenges arose. Agreements had to be reached on the value of the infrastructure-related resources (e.g. payroll management, training budgets, research and development activities) that partner organisations contributed to a pooled budget. However, it was difficult to dis-aggregate those aspects of the infrastructure that related to the services now delivered by the partnership, without destabilising support for the remaining functions of the partner organisation.

> It's all the non-cash services we provide ... but we still do the payroll for [the rest of] our staff, we provide training for the social services staff, we provide contract support.

Difficulties also arose in deciding the proportions of any national increases in NHS and local authority budgets that should be contributed to a pooled budget; these difficulties were increased when NHS and local government received different percentage increases.

> The local authority would only guarantee year on year to put in the same amount of cash … They've just had their third year of a standstill budget … the health contribution to the pool is going up and the local authority, in real terms, is shrinking.

When these national budget increases were used to fund across-the-board inflation-linked pay awards, one partner could feel it was subsidising the other who had not been able to contribute the full increase. It could also be difficult to persuade NHS partners that new 'growth' money should be contributed to the pool and spent on unspecified health and social care services, rather than on health services alone. User charges for social, but not health, services also had implications for the management of a pooled budget if the volume of services that attracted charges expanded or contracted, thereby affecting net (but not gross) expenditure.

Most partnerships were funded from a combination of mainstream budgets and 'badged' or 'soft' money, including social services modernisation grants and money to ease acute sector 'winter pressures'. While this avoided committing mainstream budgets, 'soft' money was difficult to manage within a pooled budget. It could generate inaccurate expectations about the permanent level of contributions, which were subsequently disappointed when a time-limited grant ended, and such resources usually also had to be specifically accounted for, which meant disaggregating them from the pool. Finally, pooled budgets effectively ring-fenced resources and reduced the overall financial flexibility in partners' mainstream budgets; any underspends in a pooled budget could not be used on other service areas *outside* the pool. This was most problematic in areas where one or other of the statutory partners had wider financial difficulties to contend with.

Human resources issues

In all the partnerships, closer collaboration immediately highlighted areas of duplication in the activities of health and social care staff that would lead sooner or later to changes in their roles. In a number of sites, the integration of front-line health and social care services was a key objective; however, this also presented major challenges to existing ways of working, particularly for front-line staff. These challenges can be broadly divided into 'soft' issues – culture, training and attitudes – and 'hard' issues – changes in employment terms and conditions. Strategies for tackling 'soft' human resources (HR) issues included:

- holding workshops to develop common visions and objectives
- establishing common processes and protocols across partner organisations
- integrating health and social care staff under a single management structure, while retaining existing employment arrangements; this meant devising appropriate professional accountability and supervision arrangements, for example by identifying professional leads within integrated teams
- ensuring that new staff appointments were not constrained by traditional organisational or professional boundaries
- seconding staff to a new, integrated employer before formally transferring their employment. However, this risked 'the divisiveness created by staff doing the

same job but being rewarded differently'. Moreover, any improvements in the employment terms and conditions of seconded staff could have major reper- cussions within the host agency, so secondment was seen as a short-term measure only.

The initial emphasis on the 'soft' issues of changing staff culture and attitudes sometimes reflected a deliberate strategy of generating commitment to the new partnership arrangements before more contentious employment issues were addressed. However, it was also partly pragmatic, as some of the 'harder' HR issues were difficult to resolve. For example, negotiations within central govern- ment were required to enable staff to transfer between local government and NHS employment without losing pension entitlements. Some local authorities were unclear whether their insurance policies covered staff seconded to another organi- sation and uncertainty remained about whether approved social workers could legally be employed by NHS organisations. In none of the three sites where in- depth follow-up interviews were carried out had all the processes of transferring the employment of staff to a new integrated provider organisation been com- pleted two years after the flexibilities went 'live'.

Information management and technology (IM&T)

Two types of information problems constrained the section 31 partnerships. Technical problems included hardware and software incompatibilities, incompati- bilities between coding systems and standards, incompatibilities *within* local government and NHS organisations, and incompatibility *between* NHS and local government systems. Although non-NHS organisations should, in principle, be able to access the NHS Net, this did not seem possible in some sites. In any case, it is not possible to access the NHS Net while connected to another network, so social care workers would first need to disconnect from the local authority network. Continuing fragmentation was reinforced by the requirement to supply separate performance data for health and social services – a particular problem for social services staff who had been seconded to NHS organisations.

The second set of problems concerned confidentiality and access to data about individuals. Even where technical problems were being addressed, traditional professional attitudes and assumptions remained.

> The NHS tends to have this assumption that, to put it crudely, if you let social workers look at health records, then everyone else in the local authority will be able to look at it as well ... some of it is based on professional discrimination.

In all sites, the integration of IM&T and clarification of responsibilities for IT management and operational support had lagged behind other aspects of implementation and threatened to constitute continuing major barriers to effective partnerships.

The impact of central government policies and practice

Implementing the section 31 flexibilities did not take place in isolation and progress had been affected by national policies and pressures. Some of these wider policies were experienced as unhelpful, particularly if they appeared to prioritise different objectives to those that local partners were aiming for or if they seemed to underestimate the time and effort involved in implementation. A particular concern, given the work involved in setting up section 31 partnerships, was the expectation by central government that such arrangements should be used for relatively small amounts of 'badged' funding.

> They give us a pittance and we are asked to pool it, but it is very small relative to the whole size of the learning disability budget ... a very small tail on a very large dog.

As already noted, another problem was that national performance management and audit systems still operated as if health and social care services were discrete operations. Therefore section 31 partnerships were required to disaggregate their activities and return separate sets of data.

> The performance indicators we are required to provide to the DoH are historic, they're not about where we want to get to. We have integrated teams for older people and for adults with mental health and disability but we have to report to the DoH as if we still had separate teams. They still want us to say what's the social care bit and haven't moved to ways of judging the performance of an integrated team.

Finally, the flexibilities had not removed some of the longstanding barriers that were identified earlier in this chapter. These include the different annual financial planning cycles in the NHS and local government, and the different traditions within local authorities of contracting out both support and professional services to private and voluntary organisations, compared with the strong traditions of in-house supply within the NHS.

The impact of the flexibilities

Given the substantial organisational and cultural transformations involved in implementing section 31 partnerships, changes in patterns of services or in users' experiences were still limited. Moreover, the changes were not always clearly attributable specifically to the flexibilities – in some partnerships, respondents emphasised that the flexibilities had simply taken their existing joint strategy further.

Doing things differently

One of the most dramatic and widespread consequences of using the flexibilities was to change traditional ways of thinking about and delivering services.

Interviewees spoke eloquently of abandoning former narrow, sectoral pre-occupations, of ending a 'blame culture', of taking responsibility instead for the 'whole system' of services for their particular user group and of the recognition of their interdependence with other local agencies.

> What we are now not doing is saying 'Well that's not my problem, it's your problem'. Whatever the client's needs, it has to be solved. I don't underestimate how hard it's been to get the cultural change.

> There's less energy spent on blaming partners for not delivering and a much greater investment in maximising the use of shared resources.

> One of the good things about lead commissioning and the whole business about being joined up is that ... it has made us more outward looking and made us change our agenda. And we needed the help of social services to get us past our problems.

This was not simply symbolic. Using the flexibilities required the establishment of new governance arrangements and these provided a permanent framework for future partnership working.

> The biggest area for me is how we make decisions on priorities. With the [Health Act flexibilities] infrastructure, people automatically got together and said 'These are our priorities'. I don't think we would have been able to do that if we hadn't got the flexibilities infrastructure in place and said 'you cannot go and hide in the organisational corner'.

Contrasts were drawn between the invisibility of former arrangements for transferring resources from NHS to local authority services (under section 28A of the NHS Act 1977) and the visibility of section 31 partnerships, which moved such arrangements from the margins to the mainstream of statutory services.

> The creation of the pooled fund has acted as a catalyst and an enabling mechanism ... it has required the partners to establish robust governance arrangements and move out of traditional mindsets.

> You aren't going down two parallel decision-making processes, you're not getting different cultures. So to me it's very symbolic but it also means that you are getting a very clear message to people that we are doing things together.

One aspect of these 'new ways of doing things' was a new approach to involving users in both the commissioning and the delivery of services. As just one example, in one site the joint commissioning team had established wide-ranging consultation arrangements to inform and influence its commissioning strategy.

> We've got something like 250 individuals in the city who are directly involved in developing service models, strategies, protocols.

Meanwhile in the same site, the new integrated provider organisation had created major opportunities for users to be involved at all levels of the organisation; indeed, the high level of user involvement and perceived responsiveness of the organisation to users' perspectives was widely regarded as an outstanding early success. In addition to routine consultation exercises, users had succeeded in getting issues that were important to them onto the board's agenda.

> Often the users are kind of really dictating the pace of things and the managers are listening and responding ... it's been a two-way thing which has never happened before.

Resource and efficiency gains

Within two years of implementing the flexibilities, changes in the deployment of resources were widely reported. For example, pooling budgets had the straight-forward effect of making the process of resource allocation transparent; partners were therefore prompted to examine whether existing patterns of spending were most effective.

> The most important thing is that just by virtue of bringing the key players around the table and saying 'Right, here we have £15 million currently being spent on these services, is that the right way of doing it?'. It's an incredibly powerful mechanism.

Also, the flexibilities could improve efficiency by reducing duplication and over-lap. Lead commissioning, in particular, allowed commissioning and contracting to be streamlined and common purchasing protocols to be adopted. Then, bringing together hitherto fragmented services allowed more efficient delivery systems to be introduced. This was particularly true of integrated community equipment services that had previously been fragmented between different agencies and subject to frequent disputes over responsibilities for supplying equipment in particular circumstances; dramatic reductions in waiting times for assessment and delivery of equipment were reported.

Next, the flexibilities opened up new opportunities to access external sources of finance that would previously only have been available to one partner organisation. A common source was transitional housing benefit, which was often unknown to NHS partners; other sources included the European Social Fund, the Learning and Skills Council and the Employment Service. Finally, partnerships were able to put together complex packages of services for people with par-ticularly specialised needs, in order to save money on expensive 'out-of-area' placements. Although relatively few people were affected, the sums of money involved were not inconsiderable.

Service reconfigurations

Major service reconfigurations had not occurred; sites were approaching these incrementally, to avoid destabilising existing arrangements. Nevertheless, the flexibilities had greatly increased the options for changes, and some changes could already be seen. For example, section 31 partnerships had access to a wider range of buildings, which increased opportunities for relocating services on a more geographically equitable basis.

> The local authority is a big property owner all over the city … it doesn't actually matter that 80% of the building is going to be for NHS staff.

One way of making incremental changes was to make new staff appointments in line with future service development plans, rather than simply replacing existing staff on a like-for-like basis. People taking up these new appointments were described as 'buying into integration' and it was expected that their growing presence would help to shift the balance of staff and skills and overcome some of the cultural problems described above.

> What we want is for people from both sides, backgrounds to be able to apply for a job because they're the best person for the job, not because it's a health job or a social services job.

Synergy and critical mass

Bringing together services which had had 'Cinderella' status within their former provider organisations could create new synergy – 'added value' or 'critical mass'. This in turn enhanced staff morale, by bringing together staff who had previously felt marginal within their employing organisations.

> People feel that the organisation they're working for is an organisation that relates to what they do, as opposed to relating to trolley waits or cardiac surgery.

Enhanced morale, in turn, improved staff recruitment and retention.

> A lot of our budget was going on locums, which is much more expensive … One of our objectives was to increase the number of consultants and we've done that. I think once you start to do that you get a critical mass, then it gets easier and we're almost at a position now where we've got almost all the posts filled.

Depending on local commissioning arrangements, this 'critical mass' could generate enhanced leverage in relation to local health and social care budgets.

> It's been an important lever for improving the services. We've been trying for years … it enabled us to have various showdown meetings.

Future partnership plans: reflections on the implications of the Health Act

All the sites involved in the evaluation were positive about the role of the flexibilities, in both the short and longer terms, in facilitating partnership and subsequent integration. However, their plans for future partnership developments were heavily contingent on local contexts; there was no evidence of an automatic progression from section 31 flexibility to care trust status. Some sites wanted first to consolidate and develop their existing partnerships to a stage at which clear benefits were apparent. Others had wider ambitions to use the flexibilities for new services or user groups. One of the early sites to register use of the flexibilities had decided to nest its extensive use of section 31 within its LSP, with the local authority in a leadership role; this strategy had obviated consideration of the care trust option altogether. However, all sites were agreed that future plans must be developed with strong local 'ownership'.

One reason for this caution was the organisational upheaval and the absorption of very substantial amounts of senior managers' time that was involved in implementing the flexibilities. Even though the steepest part of the flexibilities 'learning curve' had been passed and the new financial and governance frameworks were available for use with other service partnerships, time was still needed to consolidate and fully implement the new arrangements. In particular, formal agreements needed time for their impact to be felt throughout all levels of the new partnership, particularly by front-line staff. Time was needed to implement both cultural and attitudinal changes, and 'harder' human resource issues. Indeed, some of these changes were still dependent on central government action.

The flexibilities were also being implemented against a background of wider organisational upheaval. The evaluation was completed just as the remaining PCGs became PCTs and took on the responsibilities of the former health authorities. As subcommittees of their health authorities, PCGs did not have the legal status to be full partners in using the flexibilities, although many sites did note their involvement as non-signatory partners. Moreover, in some sites new PCTs were created from the merger of the former PCGs. These changes demanded attention to the creation of new relationships and, importantly, to securing the active commitment of a key local budget-holding and commissioning organisation. This commitment could not necessarily be guaranteed; where section 31 partnerships extended across more than one PCT, there was anxiety that the latter might want to assert a strong locality focus and introduce new, area-based fragmenting tensions into a newly integrated service.

Indeed (and paradoxically), there were wider anxieties about the potential fragmentation that could arise from Health Act partnerships. These anxieties focused on the potential of the section 31 partnerships to destabilise the partner organisations.

> As soon as you begin to pull the thread and use the Health Act flexibilities you are actually starting on a slope that moves you closer and closer such that you can't leave some [services] behind.

This was a particular anxiety for local authority social services departments if there were plans eventually to extend the use of the flexibilities across a range of learning disability, mental health and older people's services. The viability of the department and any leverage vis-à-vis the wider local authority that was derived from the size of its budget would be placed at risk.

> One of the impacts of all of this has been the gradual dawning that we were beginning to salami-slice the budgets and, in effect, the department. You slice a bit of your core budget here, a bit there, and this raises issues for the organisation.

Thus, while the early consequences of using the section 31 Health Act flexibilities appear to be largely positive, it may also be important to avoid potentially damaging impacts on broader local NHS and local government economies.

Conclusions: the implications for care trusts

This chapter has outlined the very real challenges – structural, financial and cultural – involved in bringing health and social care services together within a single organisational structure. Many of these challenges will also characterise the establishment of care trusts. However, the evaluation of the section 31 flexibilities has also demonstrated the vital importance of three factors.

1 Implementation requires strong, visible leadership and commitment to the new partnership arrangements. Senior managers with previous histories of working together, with a consequent legacy of substantial levels of trust, and who now have sufficient time to devote to overcoming the many practical difficulties involved in integrating organisations and services, are vital. It is their ways of thinking that are most immediately transformed by the new opportunities for integration; this experience will need to be communicated to managers and front-line professionals at all levels in the partner organisations.
2 Implementing integration takes time. The section 31 flexibilities offer no 'quick fix' to the difficulties of collaboration and neither, therefore, will the creation of care trusts. Time is needed for partnerships to develop effectively, to reconfigure services and, ultimately, to transform the experiences of service users. Moreover, organisational turbulence, the absorption of substantial amounts of senior managers' time and the cultural changes demanded of front-line staff all represent substantial initial costs. It remains to be seen whether such resource-intensive structural reorganisations can ultimately deliver better services and improved well-being for those who use them.
3 It is by no means the case that using the section 31 partnership flexibilities is necessarily simply one step along an inexorable road to care trust status. The ways in which the section 31 flexibilities can facilitate partnership and integration, and the precise organisational and governance forms which that integration takes, will depend upon local histories, priorities and circumstances.

Acknowledgement

The research on which this chapter draws was funded by the DoH. However the views expressed are those of the authors alone.

References

Audit Commission (1986) *Making a Reality of Community Care.* HMSO, London.

Clarke J and Glendinning C (2002) Partnership and the remaking of welfare governance. In: C Glendinning, M Powell and K Rummery (eds) *Partnerships, New Labour and the Governance of Welfare.* Policy Press, Bristol.

Department of Health (1998) *Partnership in Action.* DoH, London.

Glendinning C (1998) Health and social services for frail older people in the UK: changing responsibilities and new developments. In: C Glendinning (ed.) *Rights and Realities: comparing new developments in long-term care for older people.* Policy Press, Bristol.

Glendinning C, Hudson B, Hardy B *et al.* (2002) *National Evaluation of Notifications for Use of the section 31 Partnership Flexibilities of the Health Act 1999: final project report.* National Primary Care Research and Development Centre/Nuffield Institute for Health, Manchester/Leeds.

Hudson B and Henwood M (2002) The NHS and social care; the final countdown? *Policy and Politics.* **30**(2): 153–66.

Hudson B, Young R, Hardy B *et al.* (2001) *National Evaluation of Notifications for Use of the section 31 Partnership Flexibilities of the Health Act 1999: interim report.* National Primary Care Research and Development Centre/Nuffield Institute for Health, Manchester/Leeds.

Hudson B, Young R, Hardy B *et al.* (2002a) *National Evaluation of Notifications for Use of the section 31 Partnership Flexibilities of the Health Act 1999: 2nd interim report.* National Primary Care Research and Development Centre/Nuffield Institute for Health, Manchester/Leeds.

Hudson B, Young R, Hardy B *et al.* (2002b) *National Evaluation of Notifications for Use of the section 31 Partnership Flexibilities of the Health Act 1999: 3rd interim report.* National Primary Care Research and Development Centre/Nuffield Institute for Health, Manchester/Leeds.

Lewis J (2001) Older people and the health-social care boundary in the UK: half a century of hidden policy conflict. *Social Policy and Administration.* **35**(4): 343–59.

Means R, Morbey R and Smith R (2002) *From Community Care to Market Care?* Policy Press, Bristol.

Nocon A (1994) *Collaboration in Community Care.* Business Educational Publishers, Sunderland.

Wistow G and Hardy B (1996) Competition, collaboration and markets. *J Interprofessional Care.* **10**(1): 5–10.

CHAPTER 3

The Somerset story: the implications for care trusts of the evaluation of the integration of health and social services in Somerset

Edward Peck, Pauline Gulliver and David Towell

Although the Health Act flexibilities explored in Chapter 2 offer a new way for health and social care agencies to work together more flexibly and creatively, considerable partnership working was already taking place prior to the Health Act 1999. As a result, this chapter explores innovations in mental health services in Somerset which predated the Health Act flexibilities and which used other mechanisms to achieve more integrated services.

In 1996, Somerset Health Authority and Somerset County Council issued the findings of a review of mental health services which catalogued a series of problems that would have been familiar to most localities around England at that time. However, the response of the health authority and county council to this report was without precedent. They decided to introduce joint commissioning through the establishment of the Joint Commissioning Board (JCB) and integrated provision through the creation of the Somerset Partnerships Health and Social Care NHS Trust (the Trust) simultaneously on 1 April 1999. Almost as unusually, the two agencies also commissioned an evaluation of the impact of these innovations during the first 30 months from the Centre for Mental Health Services Development, Kings College London. This chapter summarises and then reflects upon the findings of this evaluation. The aims and methods of the evaluation are summarised in Box 3.1. A more detailed account of the methodology – and indeed of the findings – is presented in Peck *et al.* (2002).

The structure of the innovation in Somerset

Before presenting the findings of the research, it is important to be clear about the structure of the innovation in Somerset. The JCB was a sub-committee of both Somerset Health Authority and Somerset County Council, with the power to take

---

Box 3.1   Aims and methods of the evaluation

Aims
To identify the impact of joint commissioning and combined service provision through:

- identification of the impact of the changes on service users and carers
- assessment of the impact of changes on the professional staff involved
- identification of aspirations and beliefs of the agencies involved for joint commissioning and joint provision of mental health services in Somerset, and how these changed over time.

Methods
Each of the following data collection methods were implemented annually – once immediately prior to the integration and in the two years immediately after the integration:

- structured interviews with service users, incorporating the Lancashire Quality of Life Questionnaire, the Camberwell Assessment of Need Scale and the Verona Service Satisfaction Scale
- focus groups with self-selected service users and their carers
- a self-administered survey of all staff members involved with adult mental health service provision
- exploratory workshops with self-selected members of staff
- semi-structured interviews with senior managers of health and social services
- non-participant-based observation of the JCB.

---

decisions on behalf of the two agencies. As a consequence, only the four health authority and the four local authority nominees had voting rights. The JCB never possessed any pooled budgets as the two sub-committees continued to exist within the JCB, each responsible for resources committed by their own agency, albeit against a shared specification. The complete membership of the JCB, and the status of those members, are presented in Box 3.2. A number of additional county council and health authority personnel attended regularly, so much so that they were also given nameplates; at the meeting in June 2001, there were 24 nameplates around the table.

Box 3.2   Membership of the JCB in July 2001

- Somerset Health Authority × 4 – 2 executives, 2 non-executives – voting.
- Somerset County Council × 4 – 4 elected members – voting.
- Primary Care Trusts × 4 – non-voting.
- Users × 2 – non-voting.
- Carers × 2 – non-voting.
- Combined Trust × 2 – 1 executive, 1 non-executive – observing.

The Trust became the first NHS provider organisation in England to employ and manage staff – around 120 – transferred from a local authority social services department. It also took over responsibility for facilities and budgets previously under the auspices of that authority. About 20 approved social workers under the Mental Health Act 1983 remained in the employ of Somerset County Council, outposted to the Trust. The integrated Trust had a total income of nearly £30 million in 1999–2000, of which around roughly 10% came from the county council. In recognition of the social care responsibilities of the Trust, a director of social care filled the discretionary position on the Trust board. At the outset, the major priorities of the Trust were: to introduce locality management arrangements; to integrate care management and the care programme approach (CPA); and to co-locate health and social care staff. At the same time, the Trust had to address an annual financial deficit of approximately £500 000.

By 1999, many localities in England had adopted joint commissioning between health and social services, and the DoH had issued guidance on the topic in the mid-1990s. This aspect of the innovation was not, therefore, that unusual. However, the establishment of the JCB alongside the creation of the integrated Trust made the approach to partnership in Somerset unique.

The governance arrangements adopted in Somerset differed from those available to care trusts in a number of respects. First, and fundamentally, the Trust was a traditional NHS trust of 11 members, without the extended local authority representation present on a care trust board. However, and apparently giving balance to the arrangements, the local authority possessed half of the voting places on the JCB, whilst contributing only a small proportion of the commissioning budget. Second, the JCB exercised its authority by regularly calling the Trust to account, effectively combining the decision-making processes around commissioning and providing in one forum to such an extent that questions were frequently raised about the role and function of the Trust board.

The origins of the innovations

What was it about Somerset that led it to take this unique comprehensive approach? In order to answer this question, it is necessary to look at the origins of the innovations in Somerset. One retrospective account from Somerset (Somerset Health Authority and Somerset Social Services, 1999) lists the 'positive influences' (p 6) that facilitated the innovations in Somerset (see Box 3.3). During interviews, local participants cited the importance of long-standing shared boundaries leading to trust being created amongst a networked elite without major ideological differences. A recent history of successful joint initiatives and a lack of operational pressures, combined with little tradition of dissenting trade unionism amongst a largely static workforce were also seen as relevant. The Partnership Readiness Framework (see Chapter 1) is one way of looking at the key ingredients for effective partnership. At the start of the research, Somerset appeared to the authors to possess all of these characteristics (and a few more helpful ones besides).

At the time of writing, almost four years after the creation of the JCB and the Trust in Somerset, many localities have still not achieved this combination of joint commissioning and integrated provision. Still fewer have replicated the model of

---

Box 3.3   The positive influences in Somerset

- A history stretching back many years of health and social services working closely together – the learning difficulties strategy which had lasted 10 years and resulted in the closure of all the learning disability hospitals and the transfer of responsibility for service delivery (involving the transfer of health authority funding) across to Social Services for all those people except where there were clearly defined health needs.
- Co-terminous boundaries which made negotiation and reaching agreement that much less complicated.
- The fact that the service was conceptualised from the 'bottom-up' with each step being in response to consideration around the delivery of good quality care made it easier to gain staff support for changes.
- The detailed consideration of the issues to be tackled before reconfiguration took place rather than after.
- 100% commitment from both the Chief Executive in the Health Authority and the Director of Social Services, which gave the support and leadership to other staff to take whatever steps were necessary to achieve desired goals.
- The fact that we did not seek to save money but to ensure the best possible service for the funding available again generated support from staff.
- A sense of partnership and openness with individuals willing to give up some of their 'authority', and a sense of ownership of other people's problems.
- The government ethos of working in partnership as opposed to a very rigid purchaser/provider relationship.

Somerset Health Authority and Somerset Social Services, 1999

---

integration of provision (transfer of employment), preferring to second social care staff to the NHS provider. This suggests that the circumstances in Somerset were unusual. Advocates of the Somerset approach argue that these 'seconded' arrangements do not constitute genuine integration and are merely the first step in a process which will lead inevitably to staff transfer in due course.

The alternative argument suggests that the key aspect of integration is the creation of single line management arrangements for health and social care staff, and does not need any change of employer. Indeed, such a change may be disruptive, both for services (e.g. around staff retention) and for individuals (e.g. around pension arrangements). As a consequence, 'secondment' and other approaches may deliver the desired outcomes as well as, if not better than, the Somerset model, at least in the short term.

This is often a central debate in the local decision about whether to pursue care trust status. Within a care trust, it is assumed that social care staff will transfer their employment to the NHS, either at the outset or soon thereafter. The evidence from Somerset on the extent to which the innovations there, in particular the creation of a single employer, have delivered the benefits envisaged at their inception is obviously important to this debate. It is to discussion of this point that this chapter turns next.

Somerset prior to integration

Immediately prior to the integration, during the first round of data collection in March 1999, service users reported being generally happy with the services received, although they expressed some concern about their relationship with some staff members (e.g. perceived lack of respect). In addition, they were generally dissatisfied with inpatient services.

Ahead of the innovation being implemented, Somerset staff members (at least those who completed the questionnaire) were comparable with a nationwide sample (Onyett *et al.*, 1994) of mental health staff with respect to their role clarity, job satisfaction and morale. Despite government exhortations promoting joint working between health and social services being in place for over 25 years (e.g. DHSS, 1975), and community mental health teams (CMHTs) becoming common in England during the 1980s (Sayce, 1989), members of staff appeared to associate more with members of their own profession than the national sample, perhaps partially as a consequence of CMHTs not having been created across most of Somerset.

Before the introduction of the changes, senior managers and members of the JCB were positive about the envisaged impact of the integration. They suggested that it had the potential to bridge the cultural divide between health and social services staff members, and create a seamless service for service users.

Somerset after integration

The following sections summarise the key findings of the research at its completion in July 2001, presented first in relation to service users, then staff, JCB members and also carers.

Service users

- Between 1999 and 2001, there was a decline in the proportion of service users who reported that they had problems keeping themselves occupied and who indicated that they needed more to do with their leisure time. There was also an increase in the proportion of service users who were positive with regard to their self concept between 1999 and 2001.
- Service users reported that mental health services helped them to feel secure and supported, although concern was expressed throughout the evaluation about the experience in inpatient settings and about the attitude towards users, and the availability, of some staff.
- In 2001, a number of service users indicated that the services provided by Somerset Partnerships Trust were better co-ordinated than previously. However, concern was expressed that groups have become more limited as buildings were turned into offices for co-located teams, and some had, or were believed to be about to be, closed.
- A small number of service users reported that their engagement with the service had helped to increase their independence and get them back into society.

- There was a concern expressed by service users throughout the evaluation that no alternatives had been provided to admission to hospital in crisis.
- Some service users reported that negotiation of care plans had failed to become consistent practice and was largely dependent on the staff member that they were involved with.

Overall, the findings suggested that there had been improvements in the mental health status of many of the services users interviewed. These improvements may not have been solely related to the implementation of the review, although they were delivered during a period of major organisational change. However, by 2001, service users had become more positive about the services they were receiving. Initiatives were put in place by senior management to encourage service user involvement in the design of mental health services – at both an individual and service level – but local support for these was inconsistent. Practical issues concerned with the availability and attitudes of staff, and access to buildings, continued to exercise local users more than strategic issues.

Staff

- There was a worsening of all quantitative indices measuring job satisfaction, role clarity and morale immediately after the integration. However, two years after the integration, the majority of these indices had stabilised and, in some cases, there were minor improvements.
- Three main themes were present in the data: organisational identity, role clarity and inter-disciplinary working, and leadership and management. Some staff members were troubled by a perceived lack of identity for the Trust, discomforted by the potential for changed relationships with colleagues and disgruntled with the management structure in relation to the expectations placed upon locality and team managers, and their perceived lack of preparation for these roles.
- Work overload was a major cause for concern for many staff members. Workload was perceived to have increased since the integration as a result of some staff members reportedly being moved into management positions without replacement and a reported increase in bureaucracy and reduction in therapeutic time due to the implementation of the combined CPA and care management process.
- Numerically small disciplines within the Trust displayed a high level of anxiety over whether their views were represented and/or acknowledged at the Trust management level.
- There had apparently been some improvements in team environment, with the closer vicinity of colleagues improving relationships and communication. In addition, some staff members reported that they were able to pick up new skills and knowledge from their new colleagues. However, boundaries between professionals continued to exist within community teams, and between these teams and other services, especially inpatient services, which felt largely excluded from the integration.

The staff survey revealed that there was a reduction in job satisfaction, morale and role clarity between 1999 and 2000. By 2001, these reductions were levelling-off and in some cases reversing. Some staff members were beginning to adjust to being managed by a manager from another discipline and were appreciating the opportunities for service delivery and personal learning presented by co-location with other disciplines. Concerns continued, however, about the capacity and capability of locality and team managers to deliver change in the devolved management structure without the introduction of personal and organisational initiatives. Further, there were some concerns about the apparent ambition of some individuals within the Trust and the JCB to create a 'shared culture', sometimes interpreted by staff as a threat to professional identity.

JCB members and senior managers

- The main role of the JCB, as described by its members, was considered to be 'cementing the partnership' between health and social services.
- There were doubts expressed by JCB members about whether the JCB was fulfilling the roles outlined in its constitution (to commission, monitor and evaluate mental health and social care services in Somerset). Those members who expressed such doubts indicated that 'much of the horse trading' for commissioning of mental health and social care services was done elsewhere, leading to user and carer members of the JCB questioning their level of involvement in the decision-making process.
- PCGs and PCTs were considered by many of the senior managers and members of the JCB to have the potential to have a significant impact on the decision-making process in the JCB. However, there was also an acknowledgement that there was a lack of preparation for the involvement of primary care. As a result, there was uncertainty expressed by the primary care representatives about their role in the JCB.
- Questions were raised about the contribution and accountability of the Trust in the delivery of the aspirations for integrated provision, in particular the creation of a sense of identity for the new organisation. Although JCB members acknowledged that 'we did it, so that has to be the biggest achievement', towards the end of the evaluation discussions began to revolve around whether the Trust knew 'what sort of organisation it was', or if it was 'reactive and crisis driven'. This reflected a concern that the integration itself had become the overriding priority, relegating other objectives of the original review.
- Many of the aspirations of JCB participants for the integration were framed in terms in changes of 'culture', but questions remained about the nature of the changes required, and thus the extent to which they had been, or could have been, achieved. JCB members reported that, within the Trust, cultural differences did not just relate to the integration of health and social services, but also to professional boundaries and moves to a devolved management style. However, when prompted on what activities could be undertaken to facilitate these changes, there was an acknowledgement that 'we realised that we are not going to solve that issue without actually living together'. Implementation of locality management and co-location of staff largely constituted the organisational development programme within the Trust, which it was anticipated would address these issues.

- Despite being given relatively favourable financial settlements, in 2000/01 in particular, the Trust failed to overcome its underlying revenue problems during the study period.

Overall, the implementation of the review in Somerset built upon and enhanced the established positive relationships between executive and non-executive directors within Somerset Health Authority and officers and members within Somerset County Council. The emergence of PCTs suggested profound potential consequences for both the structure, but more importantly the process, of decision making in Somerset, but during the study period these interests were incorporated into the existing structure and process. However, the ways of making decisions in Somerset – both in and around the JCB – restricted effective user and carer involvement.

Carers

Data were also collected from annual focus groups with carers. They revealed the following themes:

- There was some evidence of perceived improvements in service delivery in the Trust. These improvements included the co-ordination of service delivery, the appointment of permanent consultants, and, in some cases, increased communication with staff members.
- Problems continued to exist, however, with the identification, involvement and provision of information to individual carers.
- The carers aspired to 'real' involvement in the treatment of those who they care for, such as being told of the contents of a care plan and being informed when changes were made to the services provided.
- There was some evidence that good practice in relation to carer involvement existed within the practice of individual key workers; however, this experience was not yet sufficiently consistent and carers acknowledged that these experiences were attributable to the individuals involved.
- Some carers reported that Trust staff members required further understanding of the needs of the family who were helping to care for a service user.

There was an indication that some carers felt that there had been improvements in service delivery; however, for others the impact of the integration was not as obvious. Problems continued to exist around the identification and involvement of carers in services, both at an individual and a county-wide level. The carers reported staff members should be encouraged to have a better appreciation of the role of the carer in supporting service users.

Discussion

Somerset introduced two major innovations, joint commissioning and integrated provision, without apparently reducing the quality of services. To some extent this achievement reflected the continuity within the system: the continuity of decision-making approaches within and around the JCB, the continuity of personnel in locality and team management, and the continuity of practitioners. Towards the end of the evaluation, there was some concern emerging that further change was perhaps being impeded by this degree of continuity. It was the new elements, in particular the integrated Trust and the multi-disciplinary community teams, which struggled most to establish an identity.

The JCB seemed to participants to make at least three important contributions to the local system. First, it was the forum within which inter-agency partnership was publicly enacted. Second, it was the vehicle for sustaining the commitment to mental health of senior players. Third, it brought added elements of openness and public accountability to the commissioning and providing of health and, to a lesser extent social, care. Clearly, these contributions could not have been made without its creation. However, it is important to acknowledge that these contributions were as much symbolic (i.e. in the fact of its existence) as in the nature of the decisions that it took.

In contrast, the establishment of the combined Trust did not appear, by the conclusion of the evaluation period in July 2001, to have delivered any significant benefits that had not been delivered elsewhere in England without the transfer of social care staff to NHS employment. This is not to say it did not achieve change (e.g. improved care co-ordination within co-located teams). However, there is no way of knowing whether comparable change would have been achieved in Somerset without the combined Trust, although it is arguable that the acknowledged quality of leadership within the Trust would not have been attracted without the novelty of that combination. Nonetheless, the personal and organisational development approach adopted in Somerset was insufficient to overcome the problems around staff identity and professional culture that were apparent from the outset.

The findings in Somerset concerning the Trust are consonant with many of the findings from private sector research on mergers and acquisitions. In a review of this literature, Field and Peck (forthcoming) suggest that the evidence provides a good indication of what to expect when health and social care organisations integrate:

- that strategic objectives are achieved only infrequently
- financial savings are rarely attained
- productivity initially drops; staff morale deteriorates
- there is considerable anxiety and stress amongst the workforce.

Similar conclusions are drawn by Fulop *et al.* (2002) from their study of NHS trust mergers in London. Further, as an earlier review (Cartwright and Cooper, 1994) contends, many of the problems in the private sector arise as a consequence of contrasting cultures in the merging organisations. In these circumstances, the creation of the Somerset Trust may be viewed as a qualified success; all of these elements were present to some extent, but none to the extent that crises, e.g. in terms of increased numbers of serious incidents or in decreased staff retention, occurred. Finally, Field and Peck (forthcoming) identify from the business world and public sector plenty of good advice on how to manage the merger process (books, e.g. Feldman and Spratt, 1999; Marks and Mirvis, 1998; booklets, e.g. Coopers and

Lybrand, 1993; Health Education Authority, 1999; and articles, e.g. Carey *et al.*, 2000; Kroll, 2000). These may repay attention from health and social care managers, albeit that they seem to have made little impact on their private sector counterparts.

It is also important that the achievements in Somerset are put in the context of studies of implementation. In their seminal study, Pressman and Wildavsky (1973) reflect on the widespread failure of implementation of innovations: 'if we thought from the beginning that they were unlikely to be successful, their failure to achieve stated goals or to work at all would not cry out for special explanation' (p 87). Widespread failure is a theme in many studies of implementation (e.g. Barrett and Fudge, 1981; Marsh and Rhodes, 1992). Against this backdrop, the progress made in Somerset between January 1999 and June 2001 appears more to be as a cause for congratulation than a cause for concern.

A post-script to the research

One of the concerns of the authors was always that 30 months was too short a period to see the long-term benefits that might emerge from integration. In the summer of 2002, the first author returned to Somerset to discuss developments. Three major themes emerged which, although not supported by the strength of data of the original research, do seem illuminating.

1 The Trust was starting to deliver service improvements which were either proving elusive elsewhere (e.g. an integrated health and social care electronic patient record) or piloting new initiatives (e.g. direct payments for users consisting of both health and social care resources). These did appear to be important benefits of the integration which had not been achieved elsewhere in England.
2 The JCB had been subsumed into a multi-client group commissioning board in April 2002 upon the creation of an LSP and the establishment of four PCTs in Somerset (and the dissolution of the health authority). Being innovative – and held up as a national model of good practice in *The NHS Plan* (DoH, 2000) – did not protect the JCB from the broader changes within the health and social care system.
3 The underlying financial problems of the Trust, which had been ameliorated by the investment of the JCB up to March 2001, started to become clearly apparent during 2001 and 2002. Vacancies were removed from establishments, buildings were closed in a process of service re-design and the warm breath of the new StHA was increasingly felt on the neck of the Trust. The small revenue base of the Trust started to become an issue and its future as a stand-alone organisation began to be discussed. In these circumstances, it is perhaps surprising that the option of transforming the Trust into a care trust was not pursued; a not unfamiliar example, maybe, of an early innovator being unable to respond to a changing context.

Conclusion: the lessons for care trusts from Somerset

So, finally, what are the lessons for care trusts from the Somerset experience? These are summarised in Box 3.4.

Box 3.4   The key messages from Somerset

- Be realistic about what can be achieved given the local history and context (*see* Box 3.3).
- Be mindful of the balance between change and continuity in the new system.
- Be careful in the articulation of aspirations in respect of 'culture' and in particular avoid ambiguity that may create staff anxiety.
- Be creative in the design of personal and organisational development programmes that support managers and teams.
- Be inclusive and ensure that all elements of the service, including inpatient care, can see a benefit from integration.
- Be careful that important objectives are not overlooked in the focus on integration itself (it is the means, not the end).
- Be prepared for certain things to get worse before they get better.
- Be ready for the changes to take three to five years to start to bear the fruit that current arrangements have not.

More importantly, perhaps, the experience in Somerset highlights again the relevance of the Partnership Readiness Framework (*see* Chapter 1). The successful creation of care trusts, or their equivalents such as the Somerset Trust, has to be the structural outcome of effective partnerships. The agreement of consenting agencies based on the history of a trusting relationship appears essential. Voluntarism seems to be a key feature, but voluntarism is not enough. After all, agencies behind one of the first tranche of care trusts are reported to have tried to use this structural solution to solve longstanding inter-agency problems only to find that these have been largely inherited by the new agency. The Somerset story suggests that both positive history and informed consent will need to be on the side of care trusts if they are to succeed in delivering the desired outcomes. Without these features, the creation of care trusts will merely move old problems to a new setting.

Acknowledgements

This study was funded by Somerset Health Authority and Somerset County Council and they wished the site of the study to be revealed. The views expressed are those of the authors and not necessarily those of the funding bodies.

References

Barrett S and Fudge C (1981) Examining the policy-action relationship. In: S Barrett and C Fudge (eds) *Policy and Action*. Methuen, London.

Cartwright S and Cooper C (1994) The human effects of mergers and acquisitions. In: C Cooper and D Rousseau (eds) *Trends in Organizational Behavior* (volume one). John Wiley and Sons, London.

Carey D, Mandl A, Bohnett D *et al.* (2000) A CEO roundtable on making mergers succeed. *Harvard Business Review.* **78**(3): 145.

Coopers and Lybrand (1993) *Making a Success of Acquisitions*. Coopers and Lybrand, London.

Department of Health (2000) *The NHS Plan: a plan for investment, a plan for reform*. TSO, London.

Department of Health and Social Services (1975) *Better Services for the Mentally Ill*. HMSO, London.

Feldman ML and Spratt MF (1999) *Five Frogs on a Log: a CEO's field guide to accelerating the transition of mergers, acquisitions, and gut wrenching change*. Harper Business, New York.

Field J and Peck E (forthcoming) Mergers and acquisitions in the private sector: what are the lessons for new organisational structures in health and social services? *Social Policy and Administration*.

Fulop N, Protopsaltis G, Hutchings A *et al.* (2002) The process and impact of NHS trust mergers: a multi-centre organisational study and management cost analysis. *BMJ.* **325**: 246–9.

Health Education Authority (1999) *Healthy Ever After? Supporting Staff Through Merger and Beyond*. Health Education Authority, London.

Kroll L (2000) The race to embrace. *Forbes.* **166**(12): 184–91.

Marsh D and Rhodes R (1992) *Implementing Thatcherite Policies*. Open University Press, Buckingham.

Marks ML and Mirvis PH (1998) *Joining Forces: one plus one equals three in mergers, acquisitions and alliances*. Jossey-Bass, San Francisco.

Onyett SR, Heppleston T and Bushnell D (1994) A national survey of community mental health teams. *J Mental Health.* **3**: 175–94.

Peck E, Gulliver P and Towell D (2002) *Modernising Partnerships: the evaluation of the implementation of the mental health review in Somerset – final report*. Institute for Applied Health and Social Policy, King's College, London.

Pressman J and Wildavsky A (1973) *Implementation: how great hopes in Washington are dashed in Oakland or why it's amazing that federal programs work at all*. University of California Press, Berkeley.

Sayce L (1989) Community mental health centres: rhetoric and reality. In: A Brackx and C Grimshaw (eds) *Mental Health Care in Crisis*. Pluto, London.

Somerset Health Authority and Somerset Social Services (1999) *Mental Health Services* (report prepared for external visitors). Somerset Health Authority and Somerset Social Services, Taunton.

CHAPTER 4

Intermediate care

Nick Goodwin and Sue Peet

Intermediate care is a relatively new phenomenon but not a new idea. Concerns about meeting the needs of people who are in transition between hospital and home, or between home and long-term care, have been prevalent for many years. Community hospitals, community nursing and community-based therapists have for a long time promoted independence and worked towards preventing admission to acute or long-term care and towards facilitating discharge from hospital. What is relatively new is the increasing focus that the UK Government is now placing on the progression of patients through a range of health and social care services and the means by which it is attempting to influence the workings of this system through targeted policy initiatives.

Since the announcement of intermediate care as a policy initiative in *The NHS Plan* (DoH, 2000a) it has gained considerable prominence in the process of modernising the NHS and in improving adult health and social care services, particularly for older people. A promised investment of £900m (DoH, 2000a) coupled with a target to provide 6700 additional intermediate care places by 2004 (DoH, 2001a) have confirmed the importance of intermediate care as a prominent feature in the delivery of health and social care in the UK.

The potential significance of intermediate care is considerable for organisations, professionals and individuals within the health and social care system. Implementation of intermediate care policy requires a substantial rethink about the culture and objectives of health and social care providers, the boundaries between organisations and the nature of financial or other partnerships between the public, private and voluntary sectors. It has raised strategic questions about the best use of human resources and, more specifically, about the roles and responsibilities of professionals. The heralding of intermediate care has sparked concerns about access to appropriate skills and resources such that the quality of care is not compromised by change and that equity for all user groups is assured. The publication of *The NHS Plan* (DoH, 2000a) and the *National Service Framework for Older People* (DoH, 2001a) has elicited a range of responses from the enthusiastic, to the cautiously welcoming, to the seriously concerned. The implementation of intermediate care policy is a significant case example of the redesign of health and social care provision and lessons from its development are likely to have resonance for emerging care trusts. Fundamentally, the success of intermediate care depends on the re-modelling of a range of partnerships between acute care and community care, health and social care, and public and independent provision.

Intermediate care in context

In the second half of the twentieth century the delivery of healthcare for older people within the NHS underwent a significant transformation. Shorter overall length of stay and the reduction in long-stay beds for older people provided impetus to the management of patient flows through the system in the most efficient and cost effective manner possible. In 1997, the Audit Commission published *The Coming of Age*, a report that examined the efficiency and effectiveness of continuing care and community care services for older people. This report provided evidence to support the generally held belief that there were increasing pressures being put upon acute services within the NHS, particularly as a result of an increase in emergency medical admissions amongst older people. The Commission also reported that the proportion of people aged 75 years and over having a hospital inpatient episode each year had increased from 13% in 1982 to 18% in 1994.

The Audit Commission expressed its concern about the reduction of rehabilitation resources, which it felt had the detrimental effect of limiting options for recovery available to the NHS (Audit Commission, 1997). It described a vicious circle in which pressures on hospital beds were increasing, leading to patients being discharged earlier. This in turn was resulting in more people receiving expensive residential and nursing home care. At the same time, there were insufficient levels of rehabilitation services to promote effective recovery for those patients who needed it. The Commission therefore called for better joint planning and commissioning of services. To this end, one of its recommendations was that health services should work with local authorities to develop innovative services with the purpose of reducing admissions to hospital and improving rehabilitation following treatment.

In the following year, 1998, the DoH established a National Beds Inquiry whose remit was to review capacity within the NHS and to consider implications for the following two decades (DoH, 2000b). The Inquiry, which reported in early 2000, stated that there had been an overall reduction in the national hospital bed stock from 480 000 in 1948 to 190 000 in 1998. Within this overall trend there had been a reduction in beds from 219 000 in 1970 to 137 000 in 1998/99 in acute and geriatric medicine specifically. Yet during the same period, hospital admissions had increased by 3.5% per annum between 1980 and 1994. The reason that such seemingly opposing trends could be sustained simultaneously was due to the substantial reduction in length of stay of patients in acute hospital beds, which in turn was largely driven by the increasing prominence of daycase admissions. These factors are illustrated in Box 4.1 below.

Box 4.1   Changes in per annum hospital bed use (1980–94)

- Numbers of available acute and general hospital beds fell by 2.6%.
- All admissions to acute hospital increased by 3.5%.
  - Ordinary admissions increased by 1.6%.
  - Daycase admissions increased by 12.4%.
- Length of stay fell by 3.3%.

(DoH, 2000b)

The National Beds Inquiry also reported that much of the rise in hospital admissions had been due to an increase in the number of people in older age groups admitted to acute hospital care (DoH, 2000b). This was interpreted as a possible response to the decline in community health services and the increasing pressure on GPs to care for very old, frail people in the face of an ageing population. Combined with this was the finding from the Inquiry that reductions in length of stay for older people were slowing down in the second half of the 1990s and that approximately 20% of bed day use for older people was estimated to be 'inappropriate'. For these reasons, the growth in admissions for older age groups was described by the National Beds Inquiry team as one of the 'key drivers of bed requirements' (DoH, 2000b, p 11).

The drive towards intermediate care

Since coming to power in 1997, the Labour Government has vigorously promoted an agenda for modernising public sector services. What became apparent from the findings of *The Coming of Age* (Audit Commission, 1997) and the National Beds Inquiry (DoH, 2000b) was that modernisation within the NHS depended on the ability to maintain a free flow of patients through and out of acute hospital care. Blockages in that system, such as 'avoidable' delays in discharge from hospital (of older people in particular), could be seen as impeding this flow. In turn this could have a detrimental impact on the ability of the NHS to meet modernisation targets for reducing waiting times, abolishing trolley waits in accident and emergency and putting an end to delayed discharges occurring in hospital inpatient care (DoH, 2000a). Since 1997/98, winter pressures monies made available to health authorities and trusts attempted to tackle some of the difficulties occurring during times of peak demand for inpatient care (Scrivens *et al.*, 1998). This resource was frequently used for the provision of services to prevent admission or to facilitate discharge from hospital and thus provided some of the early impetus to develop intermediate care services.

Accompanying this growing interest in managing patient flows was an increasing enthusiasm for new models of care targeted specifically at promoting early discharge and avoiding hospital admission. During the 1990s, a number of innovative approaches to older people's care explored the idea of developing new services for people with acute health or rehabilitation needs (Coast *et al.*, 1996; Hensher *et al.*, 1999). Such approaches reflected a growing belief that hospitals were not necessarily the best places to care for people with such needs. In particular, it was argued that admission to an acute hospital may signify for older people a loss of contact with family, the irretrievable breakdown of supportive mechanisms at home and functional decline with associated loss of independence (Creditor, 1993; Lamont *et al.*, 1983).

A further driver to the development of alternatives to inpatient and long-term care services has been the perception (and some evidence) that people would prefer to be cared for and supported in their own homes (Caplan *et al.*, 1999; Shepperd and Iliffe, 2003) and that those in receipt of medical care at home are satisfied with the care they receive (Wilson *et al.*, 2002). As a consequence of such drivers for change, particularly the growing policy imperative to develop intermediate care services, a very rapid promulgation of new intermediate care services has resulted.

Policy, guidance and the definition of intermediate care

The key policy initiatives heralding the arrival of intermediate care were *The NHS Plan* (DoH, 2000a) and the *National Service Framework for Older People* (DoH, 2001a). Both of these initiatives identified the development of intermediate care services as a key policy objective and an important driver in the modernisation process. The *National Service Framework for Older People* outlined how health and social care would be required to develop a raft of services targeted primarily towards older people who were at risk of hospital or long-term care admission. These would represent a 'new layer of care, between primary and specialist services' with the objectives of preventing unnecessary hospital admission, supporting early discharge and reducing or delaying the need for long-term residential care (DoH, 2001a). It was envisaged that services should provide a comprehensive, multi-disciplinary assessment and, by means of cross-professional working, aim to maximise independence and enable people to remain at or return to their own homes.

Guidance for the implementation of intermediate care has been provided by a circular to local authorities (DoH, 2001b), supported by further advice in the document *Intermediate Care: moving forward* (DoH, 2002a). Policy guidance around the definition of intermediate care (*see* Box 4.2) provided the basis upon which the reporting of investment decisions and activity plans was to be based. In *Intermediate Care: moving forward*, the DoH confirmed that the basic principles of intermediate care are that it should be: person-centred, driven by robust assessment and provided on the basis of need with full and proper access to specialist services.

Box 4.2   Definition of intermediate care

Services targeted at:

- preventing unnecessary admission to hospital
- promoting early supported discharge from hospital
- delaying or preventing the need for long-term care or continuing NHS care.

Services provided on the basis of:

- a comprehensive, multi-disciplinary assessment of needs
- an individualised care plan
- active therapy, treatment or opportunity for recovery
- maximising independence and enabling people to live at home.

Services operating:

- within a multi-professional model including a single assessment framework and shared records
- within a six week time limit (though frequently as little as two weeks).

DoH, 2001b

Its objective, the guidance stated, should be to promote opportunities for older people to remain healthy and live independently. Furthermore, it affirmed that the holistic needs of older people could only be served by a whole systems approach in which the full range of professional groups operated in partnership (DoH, 2002a).

The implementation of intermediate care has been characterised by a struggle to attain coherence in how to define it. Much of the early work which helped this process of definition came from a number of publications from the King's Fund including a very useful account of the complexity inherent in defining intermediate care (Stevenson and Spencer, 2002). At the time that *The NHS Plan* was published in 2000, a whole range of services already in operation, including community care, rehabilitation and supported discharge, had elements which shared the vision of intermediate care as well as meeting many of its stated criteria. It was therefore inevitable that the boundaries between what was meant by intermediate care on the one hand and acute or community services on the other would prove a challenge to furthering strategy and service development in this arena. The struggle for coherence in the definition of intermediate care may, over time, become simply a historical footnote as our understanding of where these emerging services fit within the wider system of health and social care becomes established. However, the quest to determine how best to apply the definition of intermediate care to service systems on the ground has been a lengthy one and it is apparent that PCTs retain different and often very broad interpretations of what intermediate care encompasses (Burstow, 2002).

What this suggests is that there has been a degree of confusion over how to interpret the requirements of this new policy initiative. In particular, much has been made of the process of 're-badging' existing services as 'intermediate care' in order to meet national targets on intermediate care beds, places and activity levels (Moore, 2002). Indeed, there are genuinely held concerns about the extent and appropriateness to which activity targets are being met. Nonetheless, these issues help one to reflect that intermediate care is not a new idea and that much that encompasses the approach was taking place well before *The NHS Plan* and the *National Service Framework for Older People* brought it to the forefront. The wider message from this is the importance of defining the shape of new service developments and identifying clearly the place they hold within the wider system of care.

The need for evaluation

Whilst intermediate care is very much 'in vogue', as with other policy initiatives the service has been emerging alongside the evidence needed to support it. The existing body of evidence has primarily examined elements of the main service models that comprise intermediate care (such as admission prevention schemes or those promoting supported early discharge). A number of these studies suggest that such schemes do not appear to adversely affect death rates, increase re-admission rates or cost more than admission to hospital (MacIntyre *et al.*, 2002; Parker *et al.*, 1999; Parker and Peet, 2001). However, a more recently published Cochrane review concluded that early discharge to hospital at home services was not cheaper than inpatient care although such schemes might offset the pressures on the acute sector (Shepperd and Iliffe, 2003). However, there is less clear evidence on community-based rehabilitation services (Parker and Peet, 2001) and, for the most part, the evidence base is not clear cut or complete. Indeed, there is some suggestion that it may not be appropriate to care for specific patient groups (such as those having experienced severe stroke) by taking them out of an acute care setting (Davies *et al.*, 2000; Kalra *et al.*, 2000). Furthermore, a number of potential problems to the approach remain largely untested, for example:

- the potential that the existence of admission avoidance schemes might fuel demand
- the possibility that some groups of patients who do not get admitted to hospital may be more at risk while cared for at home and that their conditions may become exacerbated, hence necessitating an admission at a later date
- that promoting discharge to home may potentially move patients before they are stable, hence risking deterioration in their health
- that intermediate care may increase workload and the burden on GPs or primary care.

As a result of these unknowns, those charged with the responsibility of implementing intermediate care have been described as 'at a frontier beyond the comfort zone provided by the evidence base, with researchers playing a game of "catch up and evaluate" in their wake' (Carpenter *et al.*, 2002, p 97). Indeed, health and social care organisations have progressed with some caution since they have had to tread a fine line between getting the necessary services in place to meet the policy agenda, whilst working within the limits of what is known to be safe, effective and cost-efficient. For example, key considerations that come into play include patient condition, staff skill mix and access to specialist services for assessment, investigation and treatment. Such factors have the potential to influence whether a service can be delivered safely and to a high standard, and apply equally to both inpatient and community-based services. The debate around whether intermediate care has been able to tread this fine line sufficiently continues to be vital in the rolling out of these new services and systems of care. It also has resonance for other innovative ways of organising or delivering health and social care, including the emerging care trusts, since they must similarly develop within uncertain territory.

Evaluating intermediate care services for older people: lessons for care trusts

Since the evidence base for intermediate care remains relatively underdeveloped and particularly since intermediate care has moved from interesting innovation to a central policy initiative, the DoH has commissioned a national programme comprising three evaluations of the process (University of Leicester, 2002). One of these, a two and a half year research process led by the universities of Leicester and Birmingham that began in October 2001, is attempting to examine the complexities of developing and implementing intermediate care on the ground (process issues) whilst also evaluating service outcomes. The latter involves assessment of professional and service users' perspectives as well as more direct outcome measures such as physical function and quality of life at admission to, and discharge from, intermediate care schemes.

The evidence on the costs and outcomes of intermediate care schemes, however, will require several years to emerge. As a national mapping exercise within this work has uncovered, tremendous local variations exist in the method by which intermediate care services are being interpreted and provided (Martin *et al.*, 2003). Moreover, it is clear that some localities are at a more advanced stage of development than others, particularly in developing formal arrangements between health and social care staff. Despite these variations, it is possible from a range of case studies and review pieces to identify a number of recurrent themes that appear to underpin the 'successful' implementation of intermediate care (*see* DoH, 2002a; Parker and Peet, 2001; Peet *et al.*, 2002; Stevenson and Spencer, 2002; Vaughan and Lathlean, 1999). These lessons in the process of intermediate care development, examined below, appear to reflect closely the steps needed to achieve integrated care working more generally (Goodwin and Shapiro, 2001). Consequently, the process of establishing intermediate care schemes may provide many lessons to the development of care trusts.

Establishing function and credibility

Establishing intermediate care schemes has been necessarily time intensive, not only in developing the mechanisms of new service arrangements, but also in having the service accepted by local people and professional groups. Much planning and preparation time appears to be required to get things right as those organisations that commit resources to such projects are at high risk if they fail. First impressions from the Leicester–Birmingham National Evaluation's observation of intermediate care co-ordinators suggest that most activity in the first year is focused around reviewing existing provision, identifying gaps and considering how best to integrate intermediate care activities with existing services. However, as Vaughan and Lathlean (1999) have observed, the understanding and confidence gained from this process of development can lead to more trust and goodwill as intermediate care services emerge. Putting in the groundwork, therefore, is critical to success since clarity of purpose is important for teams working across organisational and professional boundaries.

The ability to think beyond existing organisational boundaries and historical patterns of service has also been important in the development of intermediate care. Given the potential of different agencies to oppose change, the presence of 'hero-innovators', or charismatic key leaders who engender trust, undoubtedly helps in establishing the credibility of schemes and in providing the drive and ambition necessary to make plans into reality (Goodwin and Shapiro, 2001; Vaughan and Lathlean, 1999). It has been stressed how strong leadership and commitment from senior colleagues in health and social care can carry forward the intermediate care agenda and persuade the less enthused to follow their lead (DoH, 2002a) and the role of 'champions' in promoting intermediate care services is gaining prominence (DoH, 2001a). It could, of course, be argued that it is not realistic to base service development entirely on the ready availability of charismatic innovators and that a strategy for promoting intermediate care should not rely on this alone. But the importance of effective leadership in championing change cannot be underestimated.

Care trusts will undoubtedly need a similar, if not longer, period of time to establish credibility amongst local people, professions and managers. Indeed, within the first care trust for older people, established in North Essex in October 2002, the consultation process was regarded as very important in creating legitimacy. In particular, for staff such as social workers, therapists and district nurses who had not worked together before, staff development and consultation was a high priority to engender support for the care trust (Griffiths and Sparrow, 2003). The lesson emerging from this experience was the need to take small steps, provide managerial support and develop positive relationships with all staff groups. A united front between senior health and local authority directors was a key facilitating factor.

Though time-intensive, the key advantage to developing some degree of collective responsibility to intermediate care (or care trusts) is to help overcome existing professional tribalism, a well-recognised barrier to integrated care working (Goodwin and Shapiro, 2001). Intermediate care requires each professional group to share (or sometimes 'lose') responsibility as boundaries in service delivery become blurred, for example by the move away from assessments led by medical staff to those that can be undertaken more generically by nurses and therapists (Vaughan and Lathlean, 1999). Indeed, the development of the single assessment process (DoH, 2002b) exemplifies the way in which traditional ways of working within health and social care are being reconsidered as part of the process of modernising services. Hence the move towards collective responsibility within intermediate care needs to be carefully handled to ensure that all professional groups can support proposed changes to working practices. The same is likely to be true in care trusts, since these require professional allegiance to a new institution and to new working practices that may impinge on existing professional pride.

Success in the development of both intermediate care services and care trusts is likely to require an approach that is grounded in the promise of better patient care rather than one that simply emulates existing professional or organisational allegiances and practices. A patient-centred approach appears to be a key element in developing intermediate care since it allows services to be redesigned to meet the needs of patients rather than vice-versa (DoH, 2002a).

Cultural change management and education

Intermediate care is underpinned by the need for partnership and understanding between agencies and individuals. This requires pro-active handling since there is a need to understand the different cultures and philosophies of professionals and managers. Indeed, the enormity of the cultural change arising from, for example, a shift from services driven primarily by management of disease to ones led by rehabilitation and prevention, should not be underestimated. Asking professionals to change lifelong working practices without investing in infrastructure to support change is also likely to fail. It has been suggested that training and education needs to be more multi-disciplinary to overcome professional exclusiveness (Stevenson and Spencer, 2002). Such issues are important considerations within care trusts since the process involves moving to a new collective philosophy about care provision.

Cultural change within the North Essex Care Trust has been described as the single most important issue in its early days. Cultural differences were inherent in the different mindsets of health and social care staff and managers. This was manifest in the different use and interpretation of language, differences of opinion on how to perform certain service tasks and managerial problems associated with merging different bureaucracies (Griffiths and Sparrow, 2003).

The elimination of the organisational divide between health and social care within the North Essex Care Trust appears to be acting as a catalyst to service integration for older people's care. For example, it was reported how the inter-mediate care agenda had accelerated since staff could no longer 'hide' behind previous organisational fences. Moreover, the potential for staff to feel lost within a labyrinthine system where responsibilities and accountabilities were vague had been tackled. Consequently, services were reported to have been successfully pulled together under the 'intermediate care' banner (Griffiths and Sparrow, 2003). Hence, it would seem that care trusts, or the creation of joint health and social care units, have the potential to facilitate the process of intermediate care development itself.

Sustainability, staffing and politics

As, historically, many intermediate care schemes came about through winter pressures initiatives, there has been a preponderance of services funded from non-recurrent grants, although this would appear to be changing as more become main-streamed. In many ways, this reflects the nature of integrated care working initiatives as a whole that more often than not are created using non-core funds (Goodwin and Shapiro, 2001). Despite the importance of kick-start funding, some of the earliest intermediate care schemes foundered due to a lack of long-term funding commitment leading to uncertainty amongst staff as to the sustainability of the schemes (Peet *et al.*, 2002; Vaughan and Lathlean, 1999). The process of secur-ing recurrent funding for intermediate care services is thus important both for the individual services and for the care system as a whole as it comes to rely upon these alternatives to acute and long-term care provision. The rise of pooled budgets, made possible through section 31 of the Health Act, may not necessarily be a pre-requisite for successful intermediate care development, but the rigour involved in such formal relationships may help to clarify organisational relation-ships. Pooled funding may also help minimise the potential for disputes and give professionals more freedom to experiment with new service models (*see* Chapter 2).

Intermediate care, like the public sector more generally, is underpinned by the need for highly committed staff. However, studies of intermediate care reveal that schemes can often be adversely affected by recruitment difficulties, for example, of available therapy staff, that are required to make up the optimum skill mix necessary. Staff recruitment and retention is a high priority (*see* Peet *et al.*, 2002) and in order to achieve this, staff need to feel valued, supported and secure in their jobs. In bringing together health and social care staff within intermediate care teams, a thorny issue has been the terms and conditions of staff associated with different pay scales, working hours and pension rights. The evidence suggests that such issues need to be approached openly and pragmatically in order to overcome tension between staff who, for example, may find themselves undertak-ing similar jobs, but working to different pay regimes (Stevenson and Spencer, 2002). It is also evident that for intermediate care services to work effectively, a well-defined management structure with clear lines of accountability is important in supporting staff operating in new team formulations (Nancarrow and Mountain, 2002).

A final key point to make about the potential success of intermediate care, and indeed care trusts, is that the national political context will play a crucial role in providing impetus and direction to such projects. As a current policy priority, the funding and sustainability of intermediate care projects may seem secure, and that should provide a positive environment for progress. However, should intermediate care be seen to not deliver the goods, then political commitment may wane. The history of health and social care is full of innovative developments that have since given way to other ideas as political commitment changes (*see*, for example, Mays *et al.*, 2001). The future development of intermediate care schemes, and indeed care trusts, will no doubt depend on changes in the national political agenda.

Conclusion

Over the coming years the national drive towards intermediate care will not be achieved without challenges since the process requires a range of conditions to be met. These include: the promotion of the concept to all agencies, the development of a clear joint vision in terms of benefits to service users and to the organisations and individuals involved, and developing a consensus that is locally negotiated. The same could certainly be said about care trusts, suggesting that the process for care trust development will be time-consuming if cultural and organisational barriers are to be overcome. However, if the process of change is handled correctly, a critical mass of local ownership and agreement to a care trust vision may enable more integrated service planning and delivery thereafter.

If the emerging lessons from intermediate care development are transferable, care trust managers will play a crucial facilitative role in keeping organisational and professional groups 'on board' as staff enter a period of instability when professional roles and functions change. The process will be of concern for all those within the changing system. Consequently, it is essential that local leaders and policy makers, at both national and local levels, are able to articulate the business case for intermediate care services or care trusts so as to engender participation and confidence. Furthermore, as Vaughan and Lathlean (1999) have found, good outcomes in terms of patient care have the potential to lead to greater support and commitment and a positive work culture.

Like intermediate care, care trusts are at the beginning of a new agenda in care provision that is focused on overcoming existing professional and structural barriers to effective care provision. This agenda is particularly focused on providing new opportunities for local agencies and their staff to tackle issues such as care provision for socially excluded groups and/or users with complex health and social care needs (such as frail, older people). The ethos of intermediate care and care trusts are strongly interlinked and their success or failure will be bound to an approach to their development that is service-led, flexible and patient-focused rather than structure-driven, rigid or imposed. A key lesson, therefore, is the need to engender local collectiveness and accountability amongst all partner agencies and individuals, in order that they may adapt working practices over time towards a common purpose.

Acknowledgements

The authors are members of the National Evaluation of Intermediate Care undertaken by the universities of Birmingham and of Leicester. However, the views expressed are those of the authors alone.

References

Audit Commission (1997) *The Coming of Age: improving care services for older people*. Audit Commission, London.

Burstow P (2002) *Indeterminate Care: the reality behind intermediate care*. Liberal Democrats, London.

Caplan GA, Ward JA, Brennan NJ *et al*. (1999) Hospital in the home: a randomised controlled trial. *Medical Journal of Australia*. **170**(4): 156–60.

Carpenter I, Gladman J, Parker S *et al*. (2002) Clinical and research challenges of intermediate care. *Age and Ageing*. **31**: 97–100.

Coast J, Inglis A and Frankel S (1996) Alternatives to hospital care: what are they and who should decide? *BMJ*. **312**: 162–6.

Creditor M (1993) Hazards of hospitalisation of the elderly. *Ann Internal Medicine*. **118**(3): 219–23.

Davies L, Wilkinson M, Bonner S *et al*. (2000) 'Hospital at home' versus hospital care in patients with exacerbations of chronic obstructive pulmonary disease: prospective randomised controlled trial. *BMJ*. **321**: 1265–8.

Department of Health (2000a) *The NHS Plan: a plan for investment, a plan for reform*. TSO, London.

Department of Health (2000b) *Shaping the Future NHS: long term planning for hospitals and related services – consultation document on the findings of the National Beds Inquiry supporting analysis*. Department of Health, London.

Department of Health (2001a) *National Service Framework for Older People*. DoH, London.

Department of Health (2001b) *Intermediate Care* (HSC 2001/01: LAC 2001). DoH, London.

Department of Health (2002a) *Intermediate Care: moving forward*. DoH, London.

Department of Health (2002b) *The Single Assessment Process for Older People* (HSC 2002/001: LAC (2002)1). DoH, London.

Goodwin N and Shapiro J (2001) *The Road to Integrated Care Working*. Health Services Management Centre, University of Birmingham, Birmingham.

Griffiths J and Sparrow S (2003) *Witham, Braintree and Halstead Care Trust*. Proceedings of the HSMC Workshop on Organisational Development and Networks, 16–17 January 2003, Health Services Management Centre, University of Birmingham.

Hensher M, Fulop N, Coast J *et al*. (1999) Better out than in? Alternatives to acute hospital care. *BMJ*. **319**: 1127–30.

Kalra L, Evans A, Perez I *et al*. (2000) Alternative strategies for stroke care: a prospective randomised controlled trial. *Lancet*. **356**: 894–9.

Lamont C, Sampson S, Matthias R *et al.* (1983) The outcomes of hospitalisation for acute illness in the elderly. *J American Geriatrics Soc.* **31**(5): 282–8.

MacIntyre C, Ruth D and Ansari Z (2002) Hospital in the home is cost saving for appropriately selected patients: a comparison with in-hospital care. *Int J Quality in Health Care.* **14**: 285–93.

Martin GP, Peet SM, Hewitt GJ *et al.* (2003) Diversity and variation in intermediate care (in preparation on behalf of the Leicester–Birmingham Intermediate Care Evaluation team).

Mays N, Wyke S, Malbon G *et al.* (eds) (2001) *The Purchasing of Health Care by Primary Care Organisations: an evaluation and guide to future policy.* Open University Press, Buckingham.

Moore A (2002) On the ropes. *Health Services J.* 31 October: 24–6.

Nancarrow S and Mountain G (2002) *Staffing Intermediate Care Services: a review of the literature to inform workforce development.* Sheffield Hallam University Press, Sheffield.

Parker G, Katbamma S, Bhakta P *et al.* (1999) *Best Place of Care for Older People after Acute and during Sub-acute Illness: a systematic review.* Nuffield Community Care Studies Unit, University of Leicester, Leicester.

Parker G and Peet S (2001) *Position Paper on Intermediate Care.* Nuffield Community Care Studies Unit, University of Leicester, Leicester.

Peet S, Phelps K, Parker G *et al.* (2002) *An Evaluation of Admission Avoidance, Early Discharge and Community Reablement Schemes in Leicester City, Leicestershire and Rutland.* Nuffield Community Care Studies Unit, University of Leicester, Leicester.

Scrivens E, Cropper S and Beech R (1998) *Making Winter Monies Work: a review of locally used methods for selecting and evaluating supply-side interventions.* Centre for Health Planning & Management, Keele University, Keele.

Shepperd S and Iliffe S (2003) Hospital at home versus in-patient hospital care (Cochrane Review). In: *The Cochrane Library,* Issue 1, 2003. Update Software, Oxford.

Stevenson J and Spencer L (2002) *Developing Intermediate Care: a guide for health and social service professionals.* King's Fund, London.

University of Leicester (2002) *National Intermediate Care Evaluation Programme.* www.prw.le.ac.uk/intcare.

Vaughan B and Lathlean J (1999) *Intermediate Care: models in practice.* King's Fund, London.

Wilson A, Wynn A and Parker H (2002) Patient and carer satisfaction with 'Hospital at home': quantitative and qualitative results from a randomised controlled trial. *Br J General Practice.* **52**(9): 9–13.

CHAPTER 5

Partnership working: a service user perspective

Diane Brodie

Introduction

Partnerships often claim to be based on a shared commitment to improving services for users and carers, and many seek to involve service users in decision making or on official boards. As a result, this chapter focuses on a different type of partnership working – a partnership not just between health and social care, but also with service users and carers. Moving beyond a discussion of involvement, the chapter looks at the example of a service user sitting on a board of an NHS and social care trust with the same rights and responsibilities as the other board members. This is undoubtedly an area that needs a strong focus if health and social care are to make radical improvements. Without drawing service users and carers into real and genuine partnerships, then improvements that matter to those in receipt of services can only be made on the basis of supposition. However this raises the question of whether a genuine partnership can actually be attained. Focusing on all the different perspectives within health and social care is enough of a thorny issue when contemplating collaborative working. So to engage with users and carers with the vision of sharing power and control really is a radical approach.

Within this chapter I would like to relate a few of my experiences as a service user who became a non-executive director on the integrated Somerset Partnerships NHS and Social Care Trust (the Trust) board. I will highlight the positives and negatives from the experience. The discussion on how this approach could have a potential positive impact on service delivery also demonstrates that, without careful consideration, many problematic dilemmas can occur. The chapter will also highlight a few implications for agencies considering a similar approach.

I have been a mental health service user for the past 11 years, spending considerable periods as an inpatient, usually detained under section 3 of the Mental Health Act for the first six years. During this time I have witnessed vast changes within the mental health system. Since my time as an inpatient, I have been heavily involved with the user movement and in trying to make improvements within the Trust, such as involvement with improving inpatient services. I set up a self-support group and was a member of a regional mental health task force. I now work in the voluntary sector for South Somerset Mind. The focus of the chapter is on my previous role, over two years, as a non-executive director for the Trust.

The Somerset experience

Somerset was already a focus of innovative work through being the first trust in Britain to integrate health and social care (*see* Chapter 3). This had been highlighted in *The NHS Plan* as an example of good practice (DoH, 2000). Somerset was now seen to be going a step further. Appointing a service user onto an NHS board, I believe, was an attempt to work in what should be seen as a 'partnership'. I was appointed onto the board on the basis of merit in the same way as all the other non-executive directors, but brought with me a background of having experienced the services first hand. I had equal responsibility as a senior manager with my fellow board members and took my role very seriously, especially as I felt my 'constituency' of fellow service users deserved a voice and had high expectations of the role.

I became a non-executive director with a mixed bag of influences. I was being sustained somewhat by an anger at a system that treats people in ways with which I disagree. I wanted something different for people who experienced mental distress. Naively, I felt my position could help challenge some aspects of the system to benefit people who still needed to use mental health services. The mental health system is sustained through inequality and the exercise of power. Individuals find themselves not only struggling with life due to mental health difficulties, but often without any voice, choice, dignity or respect. Could partnership working be a key to influencing a change to this imbalance? Given that service users are not in an equal position to exercise power, are mutual trust, respect, shared decision making and joint agreements achievable? Would this highlight that an equal relationship is actually attainable or would it just show the power imbalance as indestructible?

Fellow service users were ambivalent about my position. Some argued that the only way to make effective change was to work outside the system. Once inside you could start to become part of the system, be influenced by powerful people and lose the vision. There is also the danger, illustrated by O'Hagan (1993), that service users who share the primary concerns of planners will be accepted and supported more readily than service users who propose concerns that are equally legitimate, but which conflict with their priorities. This can lead to views being marginalised and voices remaining unheard. Also, the user movement has often been divided in its approach (Thompson, 1995, p 42):

> In the United Kingdom, its stance [the mental health user movement] is neither oppositional, given that it seeks to achieve reform through involvement in planning, nor is it wholly a partnership, given that much of its message is in opposition to the basis of the system as it stands.

This meant having to make a conscious decision on my personal beliefs. I also like the statement by Edna Conlan (1996, p 208):

> Shaking hands with the devil, but not accepting his version of events without questioning his right to define situations and to judge, is sometimes the hardest thing to do ... at least when you shake hands with the devil, you can get close enough to look him straight in the eye.

This was my starting point.

Difficulties

My appointment as a non-executive director was fraught with difficulties from the very beginning. One person suggested I should eventually move on from identifying myself as a service user and be 'just a non-executive director' whilst another emphasised that I should not forget that I was there as a service user. Therefore I had very mixed messages about my role and identity. Should I be seen as a service user being a director or as a non-executive director who just happened to have a background of having used mental health services? I felt totally bewildered.

Because my appointment was through the process of being sent an application, going through an interview process and finally being selected, I came into the role in the same way as other non-executives sitting on trust boards. My appointment was not through an election process by other service users. Personally I had mixed views on this but felt that I did not have to feel 'different' and perhaps inferior to my fellow board members through having had a different means of selection. Also, I did not have the pressure of feeling I was there as the token voice for a wide and diverse group of individuals. I may have felt more justified to be representative if I had been elected, but one person cannot hope to speak in a way that truly represents a wide and diverse group of individuals. I would support Crepaz-Keay (1996, p 185) in stating that 'the opportunity is there to air views that do not get heard either often enough or at a high enough level, the views may be my own, but they do reflect widely held concerns'.

I agree with democratic election and feel perhaps that all non-executives should be elected to their positions. However representation always seems to be a stumbling block for any form of user involvement. I feel quite angry that professionals in the mental health world are never questioned over their authority to be 'representative' for their peer group. There is never a suggestion of a democratic selection process to sit on a board or committee. To me, the same rules should surely apply. However in this instance I feel that having been appointed through the recognised process gave me legitimacy in the eyes of professionals. Personal changes that occur in terms of increased knowledge, skills and confidence, that in fact are essential to survive, can be turned against a service user in terms of their representation because they do not conform to the stereotypical image. Learning to speak the same language, understanding the jargon, is a real necessity if views are to be taken seriously. But this can challenge the professional stereotype of a service user. As Lindow (1991, p 18) states, 'people who are seen as mentally ill often feel what they say is dismissed because of stereotypes, which presume them to be irrational and inarticulate. But when these same people speak out rationally and articulately, what they say is dismissed because they clearly do not fit the stereotype of a mental health service user.'

When my new role began, the chair of the trust (my boss) suggested visiting the trust units and teams to enable me to meet as many people as possible to get an understanding of the organisation and staff. This was fine, but I had not really prepared myself for the radical difference in how I was treated. I felt uncomfortably like royalty as I was escorted around various places and introduced formally to many staff. Ironically some of them had been involved in my care previously. The contrast in how they spoke, the respect being shown (at least to my face!) and being spoken to as if I was a human being with intelligence quite took me aback. It made me reflect on the fact that a particular role very much dictates how we are treated. I was the same person as I was previously – but I was not being seen as a service user. This highlighted how much service users are discriminated against and seen as less worthy beings. Brandon (1996, p 302) highlights perhaps the unspoken:

> All of us ... claim to pursue userist ends. 'The patient/client comes first in this profession'. All of us know in our heart that is untrue ... Users are usually the last in the queue. They don't ever have reserved car park places.

Having used trust services for so long and perhaps being viewed as one of the patients who would never really recover and go back to work, I realise many staff were shocked. Most staff who had cared for me in the past seemed genuinely pleased I was now in this role. For some, it was nice to see a success story and maybe someone they could influence when problems arose in their work. Others, perhaps understandably, were very awkward and uncomfortable with me, especially when I was first appointed. It must have seemed quite bizarre to them that someone as ill as I had been was now in such a position of responsibility. Having had first hand experience of some of the practices in the trust – both good and bad – this knowledge may have seemed quite threatening in what could have been described as a power reversal.

Taking on a role of senior management brought about difficulties for my own care team in the Trust. When staff require psychiatric care, the usual protocol is to receive this from another trust. I was offered services from outside the county, but this was a dilemma for me. I trusted my team and had made vast progress with them so I was reluctant to change and destabilise myself in a period of significant change. The chief executive pointed out that although I had the choice of whether I moved to another Trust or not, it somewhat defeated the purpose of being a non-executive director who used local services. So we decided I should continue as before. Initially there was a distinctly uncomfortable feeling with the professionals involved with my care in recognition of the idea that my position could have created conflict. It could have led to the feeling that we were not able to work honestly together or that they may have been punished at a later point if something went wrong. We had to have a few meetings to ensure the professionals did feel comfortable with continuing to help me and to arrive at an agreement to discuss difficulties. It was decided that if too much conflict arose, then my care would transfer to another trust.

Initially I found some of the work as a director very taxing. Perhaps this was because I was unfamiliar with the traditions and protocols involved in serious committee work and being in a position of immense responsibility. I felt that I had to justify my presence to the other service users and help enact change, so I struggled with deciding which issues were worth challenging. I had to learn the hard way that you cannot argue every point and cannot feel totally responsible for every service user's and carer's case. Fortunately, another director gave me some essential insight into being effective, in terms of presenting my viewpoint. But often I raised questions, usually at what seemed inappropriate moments, and occasionally heated debates followed. It was a steep learning curve to recognise that, however impassioned I felt over an issue, often the system prevents any change. It was so frustrating, being effectively powerless, and knowing the effects on people receiving the service. If I was going to be part of a decision, I needed to feel it was the best one available. It was clearly the case that, as Beresford *et al.* (2000, p 194) pointed out, 'where the way one sees and interprets the world and its impact on the individual is so fundamentally at variance between two parties to a discussion, it is going to require a good deal of goodwill and a lot of patience to reach understanding'.

This led me to reflect on the role of the non-executive director within the NHS. It often seemed to be just rubberstamping a decision already decided by the executives, without much question or understanding of the impact of the decision. To me, it did bring into question how much the role has any influence, in reality, over decision making. In addition to my own personal experiences, this issue was explicitly raised in the evaluation of the Trust (*see* Peck *et al.*, 2002 and Chapter 3), which highlighted the difficulties which the Trust faced in trying to involve service users at board level and the extent to which users had any 'clout' in the decisions reached (p 12). However, this was true, not only of user representatives, but also of other board members, who themselves questioned the extent to which NHS boards were able to make decisions or were asked merely to 'rubber stamp' decisions which have already been taken (p 13). A similar issue has also been raised by the literature on user involvement in learning disability partnership boards, where there is a clear recognition that 'some participants [may] become disillusioned as they discover that real decision making lies elsewhere' (Towell, 2002).

A conflict of interests?

It soon became apparent that there was a real conflict between my responsibilities as a board member and as someone receiving the service. As a non-executive director, the role involves areas such as governance and finance. The *National Service Framework for Mental Health* (DoH, 1999), amongst other directives, was driving a non-negotiable change in terms of service delivery. Many of the priorities of service users and carers seemed quite opposed to the requirements I was expected to fulfil in this role. Campbell (1991, quoted in Thompson, 1995, p 14) suggests, 'personal experience of a system which too often fails to meet human needs and employs procedures, which leave traces of unforgotten anger and distaste leads to a deep-seated and emotionally-rooted desire for change which has nothing to do with dreams of efficiency of a cost-effective management structure'. The question of in whose best interests we were working came up so much. Was the organisation for which I was partly responsible or the views of service users and carers to take precedence?

Often I felt very alone in my position and struggled with decisions about who I could discuss certain issues with. I felt torn between the confidential aspects of decision making within the trust and the needs of users and carers. For the first year, I knew no one in the same position as myself. I was part of many user groups in Somerset and a member of a pro-active group called the User and Carer Evaluation Group, which met regularly to put views forward to the executives. At the time, this was probably the group with the most knowledge and experience about the system. However, I felt uncomfortable about what I could or could not openly discuss with them. There seemed to be a 'public face', which the Trust board maintained, and whichever decision I took seemed like a disloyalty to one or the other. I was fortunate to have a good support system from other service users and carers, and two of the executive directors. But I still felt very caught in the middle and whilst I listened readily to advice, the final decision had to be taken very much alone. Being in a very unusual and isolated position, I was in grave danger of distancing myself from either fellow service users or from board colleagues in the quest for solidarity.

Becoming a Mental Health Act manager was a role that was fraught with difficulty. Non-executive directors usually become the chair of a panel of three people, which meets once a detained person appeals against their section. This meeting consists of the panel, the professionals involved and the detained person. The managers have the power to admit or discharge patients seen as mentally ill. I will say from the beginning, I have a mixed opinion on the whole of the sectioning agenda. My own view is that being on a section and put in an intensive care, locked ward did on certain occasions keep me alive. I know how determined I felt. Fortunately, or unfortunately as it felt then, my husband at the time took action. But I am still here. I feel different about life now – at least 70% of the time anyway. So why did I struggle? I felt very awkward about being the chair of the process of looking at the reasons why people were sectioned. Often my views differed widely from the rest of the panel and I was disagreed with or outvoted. To me, if all the cases had been suicidal, clearly a risk to themselves or others, then there would have been no doubt in my mind. However, at best, this was not always the case and not in clear-cut terms. I could not see the reasoning for certain people being detained. They may have had odd beliefs, strange ideas – but sometimes it seemed inappropriate to deny them their liberty on this basis and inappropriate for me to judge normality.

I guess I was in a world of subjectivity playing at objectivity. Certain psychiatrists clearly did not like my presence or my rigorous questions. Anyway, when a young person challenged me about why she was still being detained when she only self-harmed, in similar ways to others who were not sectioned, I gave a reason – but in my heart, I did not believe it. I did not sleep that night. The next day I resigned as a Mental Health Act manager due to conflicting interests.

The role I had adopted had often been at a cost to myself and my own sanity. I was asked to be involved in a lot of areas and I was immensely busy. But always being near the edge with my own mental health, I found it impossible to detach myself and not get emotional over issues. I tried very hard not to get upset. Nevertheless, I did get emotional either because many issues were still either too raw personally or because I had such strong views about how issues impacted on many of my fellow service users. I was criticised for this, but I believe that it is when you no longer feel emotions or any sense of feeling for the people on the bottom rung – the ones receiving the service – that you might as well change jobs and deal with machines, not humans. The worst occasion for me was listening in a board meeting to the list of suicides that month. One was my best friend. I contemplated resigning at that point. Why was she allowed out, why did no one see the signs? She wanted her pain to stop and this was the ultimate method. I suppose this highlights the dilemmas of what the system could have done differently. Should power have been used to prevent her wish to go off the unit? These dilemmas are perhaps hard to solve. But I felt angry and guilty. I was part of a system that had let her down.

Key successes

In an appointment such as this it is important to be able to challenge and alter certain perceptions. My involvement gave other board members, who may or may not have a real understanding of mental health issues based on experience, opportunities to learn. As we all relaxed together more, they did ask questions and often, when a decision was to be made, they would check out my perspective. I feel it is often easy to disengage oneself from users and carers in decision making. They can be too distant, not real enough to be affected. Having a service user in the heart of the decision-making process ensures the focus encompasses the forgotten voices. As well as having objectivity, I could relate first hand experiences of how certain things affected fellow service users or myself. Certain issues can be neglected, go unnoticed or be disregarded, yet for service users they may be having a vast impact on their lives. An example of this was at a meeting discussing the issue of seclusion and what a revised policy should incorporate. Having spent time in seclusion, I spoke of my experiences and how awful this was. My perspective altered the professional view on this issue and helped to change policy as a result. The provider perspective can often get so lost in talk of strategy, finance and governance that the people in need get forgotten.

Another success resulting from my appointment was in exposing an area of bad practice within the trust. I really believe this would have remained unchallenged had I not been a service user and won the confidence of the service users involved. I knew there were problems in this particular area, but the service had no concrete evidence. My visits and chats led to one person writing to me with serious allegations. Having spoken to my chairperson, I spent more time talking, listening and building trust with the service users involved. Without betraying any of the users' wishes, this eventually led to a large internal investigation. Radical change resulted – one real benefit of having a service user on the board. A service user can talk the same language, comes from the same perspective and really can understand and empathise with other service users. This can achieve a rapport, build trust and help enact change.

Do I feel I gained anything from the experience? Yes, I did. No longer do I put people on pedestals and believe that a title gives them some special knowledge and authority. I respect people, but no longer do I believe there should be such a divide between 'them' and 'us'. My position also gave some service users a sense of hope. Many had seen me as a very unwell inpatient and could not believe the transformation. Some said if I could do it, then why not them? This was encouraging.

I also came to recognise that it was not just service users and carers who were trying to enact change. I met so many interesting people in my time on the board. It seemed that many professionals and managers genuinely wanted a system that was different. I was often quite amazed at the quite radical views of those from whom I would have least expected them. This gave me hope. Not everyone was totally sold on a strictly medical viewpoint or on a system that does not aid recovery in as positive way as it could. I had a glimpse of hope.

Sadly, my hope was lost. The Trust, like so many, ran into difficulties financially. It became apparent that services would have to be cut and units lost to other providers. And I was critical of the process (or rather the lack of it) of the decision making. A strategy appeared with no prior discussion by all the stakeholders. I was the only one to vote against it at the board meeting. I knew that this was the end – I could no longer stay on the board, look my fellow service users in the eye and say I was part of the decision to close their units. But this still left me with feelings of guilt, especially when service users and carers said that they had then lost their voice.

It is sad. Somerset could have been so different. It tried quite radical approaches that could have succeeded had more money been available. But lessons are there to be learnt. The question I have been asked is whether I would I have stayed had the financial difficulties not led to such radical cuts. The answer is yes, I believe I would have stayed on the board if the conflict had not been so great. I still feel it was an opportunity for users and carers to influence opinion and enact change.

User and carer involvement

For me, having a service user on the board had a number of advantages and disadvantages (*see* Box 5.1).

Box 5.1   Involving users on partnership boards

Advantages

- Provides a better, user-centred service by ensuring there is a focus on how users are affected by decisions.
- Promotes an awareness of what service users can offer by showing capabilities and challenging stereotypical ideas of users.
- Can raise issues that otherwise would not be thought of or deemed un-important.
- Gives a voice to service users and carers.
- Gives a positive message to other service users of what is achievable – gives hope.
- Can challenge the dominant medical perspective.
- Helps to alleviate negative language and discrimination against service users.
- Can uncover areas of bad practice when service users are powerless.
- Brings about a more holistic understanding of service users' and carers' needs.

Disadvantages

- The dilemma of balancing corporate responsibility against service users' wishes – feeling caught in the middle.
- Issues raised that hit raw nerves and emotions can lead to difficulties in coping.
- Worries of 'being sucked into the system' and losing the service user viewpoint.

- Losing the energy to challenge.
- Burnout – too much demand from the trust and not wanting to say 'no' when a user viewpoint is needed.
- Difficulty finding users to be involved.
- Still needing care and receiving care within one's own trust can lead to an uncomfortable arrangement.
- Conflicts between being a Mental Health Act manager and having been sectioned.
- Being expected to be an agent of government directives and resource cuts that conflict with the interests of users.

For agencies who are considering drawing service users or carers into a partnership position by becoming a board member, I have a few pointers.

- Such board members need to feel they are equal and to be equal.
- Such board members should not have to feel the pressure of justifying their position any more than other board members.
- Such board members should be clear as to what their role is.
- The trust must ensure the board includes people to whom users can turn for support and who can offer guidance.
- Emotional support is also essential, as such board members will often have been affected by the experiences that come up in committee discussions.
- The trust should ensure that such board members are in contact with a wide network of other users and carers for support and advice.
- Such board members should have the necessary training and guidance for their role from peers and professionals.
- Just as with other members, the views of such board members should be listened to and heard, even if they do not conform to traditional roles and ways of speaking.
- Such board members should be made to feel part of a team of other non-executives and not feel that they are different or discriminated against because of their perspective.
- The trust must not overwork such board members or put unreasonable demands on them.
- The trust needs a structure that enables wider user/carer views to be influential to the board.

Finally, it is useful to analyse my experiences in more general terms of user and carer involvement. Arnstein's (1969) 'Ladder of citizen participation' is a useful framework for assessing efforts at involving service users (*see* Box 5.2).

Box 5.2 Different levels of user involvement

1 Manipulation
2 Therapy
3 Informing
4 Consultation
5 Placation
6 Partnership
7 Delegated power
8 Citizen control

Levels 1–3 have a one-way flow of information aimed at achieving public support through public relations.
Levels 4–5 have a two-way flow of information.
Levels 6–7 lead to real participation and a sharing of power.
Level 8 leads to users controlling funds and making decisions.

Arnstein, 1969, quoted in McIver, 1993, pp 52–3

Placing my appointment as non-executive director within this ladder is difficult. At first glance, it appears to be an example of significant user involvement. However, in reality, 'placation' (where participants have an advisory role with no power in decision making) may arguably have been the case, rather than 'partnership' (where some degree of power sharing is given). To achieve partnership, Arnstein (1969) emphasises that 'this level of participation usually has to be demanded by participants disillusioned by their experiences of tokenism and non-participation, and is unlikely to be freely offered'.

In spite of some of the difficulties I encountered, I still advocate the need to work in partnership with users and carers. A lot of the difficulties I encountered could be resolved with prior planning and considered thought. If the conflicts had not been so difficult at the end, then the outcome for me could have been different. A recognition that 'at an individual level, users are more or less disempowered in their relationships with professionals unless shared decision making is actively embraced' (Brown, 2000, p 103) is essential. Partnership working could be a key to challenging the unequal exercise of power that has remained in the mental health system for too long. The dominant medical perspective needs diluting enormously if service users and carers are to benefit in more holistic ways. Certainly, bringing together health and social care in partnership is a method to challenge this strong discourse, but it still needs further robust confrontation. A new system needs developing to encompass and balance all contributions and develop services *with*, not *for*, users (Braye and Preston-Shoot, 2000).

My views may have been sought as a token gesture or for the purpose of rubberstamping a decision, but arguably, I was an equal member of the board with full voting rights. For me, the strength of the role of a non-executive director seems to relate to the individual's knowledge and understanding of the particular trust and their ability to challenge executive board members effectively. However, it also needs to be recognised that a trust board itself has questionable power in terms of radical change. Certain professional bodies hold immense power, the government is very prescriptive about the services that are required to be delivered and, if mental health services are underfunded, then opportunities for service improvement are stifled. Despite best intentions, any changes can be in conflict with the wishes of service users and carers.

But to conclude, it does appear that a radical new way of thinking is required if partnerships with users and carers are to move positively onto the starting blocks. As McCormack (1998, p 31, cited in Finlay, 2000) suggests:

> Many people forget just who the expert is when it comes to the provision of care. The professional is the person with power over resources. However, the expert is the person with the need. What balances this relationship is mutual respect between the two; i.e. the powerful with the resources and the powerless with the expertise. It is only in the context of rights that such a relationship of mutual respect can be achieved.

Acknowledgements

Thank you to Peter Hill, South Somerset Mind, and to Professor Steve Onyett, Mental Health South West, for advice and guidance on this chapter.

References

Arnstein S (1969) A ladder of citizen participation in the USA. *J American Institute of Planners*. **35**: 216–24.

Beresford P, Croft S, Evans C *et al*. (2000) Quality in personal social services: the developing role of user involvement in the UK. In: C Davis, L Finlay and A Bullman (eds) *Changing Practice in Health and Social Care*. Sage Publications in association with the Open University Press, London.

Brandon D (1996) Normalising professional skills. In: T Heller, J Reynolds, R Gomm *et al*. (eds) *Mental Health Matters: a reader*. Macmillan, Basingstoke.

Braye S and Preston-Shoot M (2000) Keys to collaboration. In: C Davis, L Finlay and A Bullman (eds) *Changing Practice in Health and Social Care*. Sage Publications in association with the Open University Press, London.

Brown H (2000) Challenges from service users. In: A Brechin, H Brown and M Eby (eds) *Critical Practice in Health and Social Care*. Sage Publications in association with the Open University Press, London.

Campbell P (1991) In times of crisis. *Openmind*. **52**: August/September: 15.

Conlan E (1996) Shaking hands with the devil. In: J Read and J Reynolds (eds) *Speaking our Minds: an anthology*. Macmillan, Basingstoke.

Crepaz-Keay D (1996) Who do you represent? In: J Read and J Reynolds (eds) *Speaking our Minds: an anthology*. Macmillan, Basingstoke.

Department of Health (1999) *National Service Framework for Mental Health*. DoH, London.

Department of Health (2000) *The NHS Plan: a plan for investment, a plan for reform*. TSO, London.

Finlay L (2000) The challenge of professionalism. In: A Brechin, H Brown and M Eby (eds) *Critical Practice in Health and Social Care*. Sage Publications in association with the Open University Press, London.

Lindow V (1991) Experts, lies and stereotypes. *Health Services J*. 29 August: 18–9.

McCormack I (1998) *Developing mutual understanding and partnership: towards a common purpose?* Conference Proceedings: the Quality of Social Care in Ireland, North and South – new perspectives, UNISON/IMPACT Conference 1997, Belfast.

McIver S (1993) *Obtaining the Views of Users of Primary and Community Health Services*. King's Fund Centre, London.

O'Hagan M (1993) *Stopovers On My Way Home From Mars: a journey into the psychiatric survivor movement*. Survivors Speak Out, London.

Peck E, Gulliver P and Towell D (2002) *Modernising Partnerships: the evaluation of the implementation of the mental health review in Somerset – final report*. Institute for Applied Health and Social Policy, King's College, London.

Thompson J (1995) *User Involvement in Mental Health Services: the limits of consumerism, the risks of marginalisation and the need for a critical approach* (Research Memorandum no. 8). Centre for Systems Studies, University of Hull, Hull.

Towell D (2002) *Partnership Boards and User Engagement: what do you think of the show so far?* Available online at www.learningdisabilities.org.uk/html/content/pftopic09.cfm (accessed 29/11/2002).

PART TWO

Care trusts

In Part One, we highlighted a number of themes and issues that care trusts will need to acknowledge and build on from our existing knowledge of health and social care partnerships. In particular, we have focused on:

- existing lessons from the partnership working literature
- the national evaluation of the Health Act flexibilities
- the evaluation of the Somerset Mental Health Partnership Trust
- the national evaluation of intermediate care
- a service user perspective on user involvement in health and social care partnerships.

However, what lessons do care trusts give us about partnership working and what has the experience to date been of front-line agencies responsible for delivering more integrated services?

Against this background, Part Two focuses on the care trust model in more detail with chapters on:

- the personal perspective of the DoH care trust lead (Chapter 6)
- common criticisms which have been made of the care trust model (Chapter 7)
- a case study from a first tranche care trust (Chapter 8)
- a case study from a health and social care community which formed a mental health care trust in April 2003, but which decided on a different route for learning disability services (Chapter 9)
- a case study of an area which considered care trust status and ruled it out in favour of other ways of working (Chapter 10).

After this, a conclusion draws together emerging themes and issues from the book and considers possible ways forward.

CHAPTER 6

Care trusts: a positive option for service improvement

Shane Giles

The opinions expressed in this chapter are those of the author and should not be taken as representing those of the DoH.

Introduction

A review of government policy over many years would show numerous national invectives to ensure that users simultaneously requiring health and social care services should receive them in a seamless manner rather than having to endure and resolve dissonant provision. Recent manifestations of steps towards that objective have included the Health Act flexibilities (*see* Chapter 2), the introduction of care trusts in 2001 and, most recently, the policy initiative around children's trusts.

There can be no doubt that the services provided in England in respect of health and social care are of a high standard, one to which, indeed, other countries aspire. They are built upon a social policy tradition of concern to ensure that those in need receive appropriate support. A major weakness, however, is that health and social care services have tended to evolve through disparate organisational structures, professional values and cultural assumptions with the consequence that users simultaneously requiring provision by both health and social care services often find themselves caught in a labyrinth of similar but differing assessment criteria, conflicting service models and inter-agency shunting of responsibility. It is these unnecessary and damaging differences that government is intent on resolving and care trusts are an important component of their solution.

Common criticisms of care trusts

Many of the commentaries on care trusts have focused on the letter and ignored the spirit of what the approach offers. Discussion has too often concentrated on care trusts being a 'structural' solution unable to resolve immediately longstanding issues such as cultural and organisational differences, pay harmonisation or governance arrangements.

Contrast this critical position with the present care trust sites (and the many other sites who have used other processes to successfully integrate services), which have found mechanisms to integrate services despite these 'problems'. These sites have made meaningful steps towards integration by taking a pragmatic view, invoking the old adage 'where there is a will, there is a way'. They have listened and responded to the views of the users of their services, their staff and the government on the need to integrate provision, and have done so effectively. While a critical analysis of government policy is, of course, essential, criticism which fails to take account of opportunities offered is counter-productive.

Change inevitably provokes concern and those in local authorities and the NHS charged with providing key services are no exception, if for no other reason than the need to ensure that the quality of provision and the integrity of services is not damaged by ill-conceived or poorly managed innovations. It was therefore right and proper that, as care trust policy was rolled out, health and social care professionals and managers thought carefully about and debated strongly the proposed model.

A significant criticism of care trusts is that they represent a take over of local authority provision by the NHS. Local authorities have a long tradition of social care provision, one of which they are justly proud, and therefore they were justified in looking critically at what care trusts would mean for these services. For them not to have done so would have been an abdication of their responsibility as the custodians of those services.

Care trusts do present a major challenge to local authorities in terms of the provision of social care services, raising issues as to the governance, planning and delivery of services. But for some local authorities, the movement towards care trusts was a logical progression of the work they were already undertaking. More than one of the present care trusts commented that they were inevitably going to form some variation on a 'care trust' – they just did not have an organisational form or legal mandate to take the next step forward until the arrival of the care trust template. The view of the local authorities that initiated care trusts, and their sister health service partners, exhibited the sort of pragmatism referred to above; a pragmatism which understands that the overriding need is one of providing relevant services to users and that debate about structural innovation as opposed to organic change or pay harmonisation may be necessary, but does not in itself deliver improved services.

It is hard to imagine that the government believes, as some commentators have suggested, that the implementation of a new structure alone would bring about wholesale service improvement. But it is the responsibility of government to lead, to be clear as to its objectives and to act accordingly. The government is concerned that the present system of provision is not as effective at it could and should be. It is not alone in that belief; representative bodies of local authorities and the NHS, trade unions, professional bodies and social and health care commentators have for a long time been critical of the boundaries that exist between health and social care. The government was therefore duty bound to introduce reform; for it not to show leadership would have been an abdication of its responsibilities.

Overall, the government remains clear that care trusts should be offered as a (voluntary) option to health and social care communities as a vehicle for service improvement. It sees care trusts as a model that may be adopted and adapted in a variety of ways. By defining a potential change through legislation, the DoH has given a clear message that significant change in organisational relationships is both desirable and possible and suggested one opportunity to the field as to a possible mechanism for carrying forward that change and improving services. But it has not given an instruction, nor has it reduced flexibility in other areas; it has simply given front-line agencies an additional vehicle to explore when considering options for service improvement.

Implementing care trusts

From the beginning, the DoH was properly concerned that care trusts should be implemented as effectively as possible and, as part of that implementation, that lessons from those setting up care trusts should properly inform the development of regulations and guidance. Care trust implementation was not to be a setting of an agenda from the centre, distant from the realities of the coal face. Rather the implementation was envisaged as a joint venture between the centre and the 'demonstrator' sites (i.e. those that would be established by April 2002).

An issue apparently regularly misunderstood is why the early sites were referred to as 'demonstrator sites'. The 'demonstration' was of the process of forming a care trust, not of the structure in itself. If that process led a locality to do other than form a care trust, that was still a positive outcome as it indicated that the site had properly considered the best option for taking forward partnership in that context at that time. What was important was that the right solution for each individual locality was established.

Initially (July 2001), nine sites expressed interest in forming care trusts at April 2002. These sites represented a diverse range of local authority and NHS bodies, commissioning and providing services for and to children, adults with mental health issues, adults with learning disabilities and older people. They apparently shared great enthusiasm in forwarding the care trust agenda – possibly surprising given that so much of the detail was then undefined.

By December 2001, some 15 sites had expressed interest in forming a care trust. By this stage, of the original nine sites, some were already looking at start dates after April 2002. Over time, the number of sites aspiring to form a care trust reduced as sites either extended the timescale over which they wished to achieve care trust status or found, for them, a more appropriate vehicle by which to integrate and improve services.

There never was a target for the number of the care trusts set by ministers or civil servants. Rather, the target was the improvement of services through the use of care trust status where it was the best model for a given locality. 'Shoehorning' a locality into this model for the sole purpose of forming another care trust was never on the agenda.

Central to establishing the care trusts was the Care Trust Network, which was a coming together of an initial 15 potential sites with DoH officials. Through a variety of mechanisms, such as email groups and national meetings, it provided communication and support between the Department and the sites, and between sites themselves. As drafts of guidance and regulations were prepared, these would be passed out through the Network for comment. Likewise, experience and expertise gained by an individual site would be passed into the Network to inform policy development and the work of other sites.

Working alongside this Network were a number of 'strand' groups, each of which had responsibility for particular issues such as human resources and governance. It is notable that these groups contained significant representation from outside of government, including interests apparently opposed to care trusts. When one now reviews the guidance and regulations there is much not of government origin; rather they display the wide-ranging processes and contributors that generated them.

The count-down to April 2002

From December 2001 through to March 2002 was a period of intense activity for those involved with the four sites wishing to be established on 1 April 2002. For the sites concerned, this involved finishing their consultations on the formation of the care trust, finalising their applications and starting to plan the changes needed should their applications be successful. This flurry of work in the field was mirrored in the DoH as guidance and regulations had to be confirmed, the applications by the four sites had to be assessed and the legal processes to establish them as care trusts completed.

The four applications, with all their associated documentation, varied in style and size, but all clearly illustrated the strong desire and a compelling case to form a care trust in their locality. It was evident that these were not the aspirations of a single individual or single organisation, but were representative of a positive view held between and across organisations as to how to develop and improve services to users.

The process for the assessment of the applications was rigorous. These applications represented the first of their kind and it was therefore essential that the fundamental change they represented was not allowed to occur without due care. It is a testament to the commitment of the applicants that all four applications to form a care trust were granted.

Early lessons

What does the experience of the early care trust sites tell us?

The emergence of the first care trusts has shown a clear appetite for the model around England. The first sites give a very clear message that, for their users, the forming of a care trust was the right and proper solution to the delivery of improved services. They tell us that the structure that care trusts offer, while not the ultimate or perfect structure, is the best presently available for the delivery of service improvement in their locality.

There has been a long tradition of bringing together health and social care services through formal and informal means. Against this background, the first care trusts have made positive decisions about forming a care trust over or in addition to, for instance, using the section 31 flexibilities or informal partnership arrangements such as partnership boards and joint appointments. The message from the first sites is simple: for them, care trusts are the right solution. It does not mean that care trusts are right for everyone, but they are an appropriate movement forward in these first sites. These sites will over time show the positives, and also the negatives, of the care trust model and will inform future thinking as to the best approach to integration as a whole. Lessons learnt through arranging governance, for example, in the care trust structure will inform the governance arrangements in non-care trust sites. There is much to be learnt from this new structure.

In addition to developing a shared vision of the way forward and melding differing histories, traditions and cultures, care trust implementation raises practical questions, such as those around governance, human resources and finance.

Health and social care agencies have traditionally had very different governance arrangements at all levels. Councillors have different relationships with their officers from those non-executive directors enjoy with NHS managers. Whilst NHS clinical governance systems and local authority best value regimes are both designed to improve service standards, they originated in very disparate circumstances and adopt divergent perspectives. For agencies forming care trusts, it is necessary to recognise that these differences have evolved over time and that each approach has strengths and limitations which need to be carefully balanced. While this is complex, bringing different ways of working together enables local agencies to take the best of their two approaches in order to ensure that they continue to provide high quality services.

The greatest asset of any organisation is its staff. The management of these staff and the use of their skills in appropriate yet flexible ways lies at the heart of ensuring that the organisation achieves its potential and delivers its objectives, and the creation of a care trust can challenge a number of traditional assumptions about the deployment of its human resources. It challenges staff by reviewing and possibly changing working practices, organisational structures and employment arrangements; all of which, without thoughtful management, could bring unnecessary uncertainty to staff and destabilise not just them, but also the organisation for which they work and the services they provide. Properly handled, however, it will lead to a stronger and more effective organisation.

Local government and the NHS are financed through very different routes, with disparate budget cycles and financial management regimes, and these do not immediately complement one another. Most importantly of all, many NHS services are free at the point of delivery while social care services may require a financial contribution from users. All these issues need to be properly understood and managed in order to ensure that public money not only secures the services it was intended for as effectively as possible, but with the high degree of probity that the general public expects. Care trusts forced localities to put in place systems that could deal with these differences and not be deflected from further integration just because these issues were hard and high-profile.

Overall, care trusts have provoked significant debate which has positively impacted upon service integration in the widest possible way. Care trusts brought to the table numerous organisations and individuals to resolve issues such as effecting cultural and organisational change and the integration of financial, human resource and governance arrangements. While the solutions reached at this time may not be final, thinking and understanding as to integration has significantly developed in the few years since care trusts were first mooted in *The NHS Plan* (DoH, 2000).

Next steps

A consequence of the debate as to the relevance of care trusts was the heightening of interest in service integration generally. Not to capitalise upon this interest would have been a wasted opportunity. With this in mind a variety of bodies – the DoH, Office of the Deputy Prime Minister, National Primary and Care Trust Development Programme, Health and Social Care Change Agent Team, Association of Directors of Social Services, Local Government Association, Improvement and Development Agency, NHS Confederation and strategic health authorities – came together to form the Integrated Care Network. The Network's objectives include: providing an infrastructure of support to front-line organisations wishing to progress integrated working between local authorities and the NHS, bringing together the wealth of experience and knowledge that these organisations have as to integration, disseminating this information widely, and using learning from the Network to inform the development of government policy.

For further information on the Integrated Care Network, visit www. integratedcarenetwork.gov.uk.

Reference

Department of Health (2000) *The NHS Plan: a plan for investment, a plan for reform.* TSO, London.

CHAPTER 7

Care trusts: a sceptical view

Bob Hudson

Partnership working – hitherto a fringe player in British social policy – was to be the fresh 'third way' in New Labour's approach to the public sector following the 1997 General Election, and nowhere was this more evident than in the relationship between NHS and social care services. In choosing this path, the alternative route of structural integration of separate organisations was explicitly eschewed. Yet within three years, the debate was dramatically re-opened by the proposal in *The NHS Plan* (DoH, 2000) to create care trusts that would combine health and social care functions in one NHS agency.

The politics of care trusts have been confusing, with the government appearing to oscillate between legislating for compulsion, and portraying the idea as simply one option amongst others that localities may wish to utilise. In reality, the proof of the pudding is in the eating and to date interest from the field has been limited and patchy. The original 15 'pilots' were soon whittled down to only nine, and it was later reported that many of the nine were likely to be delayed. What this slowness represents is a well-founded scepticism that organisational restructuring in general is not a useful activity, and – more specifically – that the costs of care trusts outweigh the benefits. This chapter identifies several reasons for such scepticism, building on arguments which have already been developed elsewhere by the author (Hudson, 2002a, b), and explores the idea of networks as an alternative model.

Absence of an evidence base

Although the first care trust projects are often referred to as 'pilots', there has been no attempt to pilot alternative structural reconfigurations, most notably one in which community health and possibly other NHS functions are returned to local authorities. Some of the evidence which is around would suggest exercising caution before opting for one particular approach. In a review of the move towards integration across health and social care, Henwood (2001), for example, concludes that:

> The development of care trusts, and the general thrust of the most recent policy direction on health and social care integration, appears to have little evidence base. An untried approach is being promoted in the absence of any clear elaboration of the model, or any exposition of

what is likely to be the best approach, for which client groups, under what particular local circumstances and conditions.

The myth of Northern Ireland

The political thirst for integrated structures is related to the apparent success of the integrated Health and Social Services Boards in Northern Ireland – a model praised by the Health Select Committee (1998) and the Royal Commission on Long Term Care (1999). In fact, recent experience suggests that Northern Ireland faces very similar difficulties to the mainland in managing health and social care pressure points, and in some respects may manage them *less* successfully. An urgent review of the provision of care in the community, and its relationship with admission and discharge practices, was commissioned by the Minister for Health, Social Services and Public Safety at the beginning of January 2000. The report identified a number of shortcomings including: services shortfalls in every aspect of community care provision, delayed discharges from hospital, waiting lists for day care and respite care, and inappropriate placements in residential care (Social Services Inspectorate, 2000). These are precisely the problems which are familiar in England and which advocates of the Northern Ireland model have argued are satisfactorily resolved by structural integration. In other words, much of the 'integration' between health and social care in Northern Ireland would seem to be more apparent than real and structural integration evidently does *not* guarantee well co-ordinated practice on the ground.

Financial dilemmas

Bringing together two different financial systems into a unified budget will not be easy. DoH guidance portrays this as a mechanical issue, much of which will already have been resolved in using the Health Act flexibilities, but this under-plays the likely difficulties. In reality, the experience of setting up pooled budgets and other flexibilities has been anything but straightforward, with disagreement over both the volume of resources and access to them (Hudson *et al.*, 2001). Commitment of large budgets to a care trust will be likely to intensify concerns on the part of local authorities, especially where they believe the care trust may 'misuse' their contribution in order to meet priorities other than social care. In particular, there will be concern that the preferences of GPs will predominate over social care interests and there will need to be some assurances that their spending levels will be protected.

In addition to these new difficulties, the longstanding dilemma of charging for social care services remains unresolved. The fact that care trust guidance (DoH, 2001a, p 8) merely states that 'the charging arrangements for local council services will remain the same' is a restatement of a dilemma rather than a resolution of uncertainty. Administrative and professional divisions arise from this financial boundary, but more importantly it impedes the experience of integrated care for the service user. From the viewpoint of the user/patient, a lack of coherence in services will continue to exist to the extent that they continue to face charges for the social care component of services.

Threat to social care values

The problems of health and social care fragmentation are not solely structural; they are also cultural. The two services have different origins and adhere to different 'ideologies', and the question of whether these can be reconciled has received scant attention. Social care sees itself as having several features which distinguish it from the approach of NHS agencies. Bamford (2001), for example, identifies three characteristic values: self-determination, participation and empowerment. These, he argues, do not sit comfortably with the tradition of medicine firmly rooted in the model of professional diagnosis and treatment, where the patient is rarely seen as an equal partner. Moreover, there is a belief and some evidence that the NHS – especially the nascent PCT system – lacks the necessary expertise in some important aspects of potential care trust activity. The Tenth Annual Report from the Chief Inspector of Social Services, for example, notes of inspections of services for older people (Platt, 2001):

> We found that the NHS was not a source of expertise about commissioning and managing social care services for older people. We concluded that in the future when PCTs or care trusts combine responsibilities for some NHS and social care services for older people, the expertise and responsibility for the social care services will need to be rooted in councils' experiences.

NHS expertise is similarly lacking in two other crucial roles: micro-commissioning and managing a mixed economy. As Bamford (2001, p 118) notes 'micro-management is foreign to health care commissioning'. Rather the NHS has focused upon large, long-term contracts with large-scale, often monopoly, providers or contracting to itself in the internal market. In parallel, monitoring of health contracts also tends towards narrowly defined performance targets, rather than outcomes for users. Social care is also far more experienced in operating within a developed and genuine market involving independent sector providers – the PCG/T tracker survey, for example, found that only three had co-opted one or more voluntary organisation representatives onto its board (Wilkin *et al.*, 2001).

In addition, Peck *et al.*, (2001) raise questions about the dubious assumption underpinning the care trust model that cultural change will occur spontaneously as a consequence of creating combined organisations or that it is susceptible to manipulation, with predictable and positive results. They ask whether the desired result is one entirely new culture, albeit comprised of elements taken from all the current professional cultures, or the enhancement of the current professional cultures by the addition of mutual understanding and respect? On the basis of an evaluation of Britain's first combined trust for mental health (in Somerset), the authors conclude (p 325) that 'this study seems to demonstrate that the creation of a combined trust is not, in itself, sufficient to create either' (*see also* Chapter 3).

Threat to democratic accountability

During the days of Conservative governments, the Labour Opposition made much of the 'democratic deficit' in the NHS, but the issue seems to have little current political status. Whereas in the 1990s, the Conservative Government – albeit reluctantly – extended the role of local social services authorities, New Labour is now suspected of plotting their demise. The political suspicion is that the care trust thrust is not about improving service delivery for users, but about central government taking control of local authority-run care services by placing them in the centrally run NHS. The political imperative behind this is the need to deliver on the NHS – to cut waiting lists and waiting times by emptying NHS beds. In effect social services are seen as a means to achieving progress in the health system, not as valuable services in their own right with different aims and objectives. Indeed, the potential local authority remit is wider than social services – the briefing paper from the DoH inviting care trust pilots also identified housing and education services as functions which could be transferred from local authorities to care trusts.

Narrowness of remit

The new partnership agenda is more complex than previously. The focus now is less upon the relationship between health and social care, than between health and local authority functions more broadly, and wider matters of governance. The trend is now towards 'multiple partnerships' in several senses:

- partnerships which involve multiple (more than two) partners
- partnerships aimed at different objectives ranging from integrated care to social and economic regeneration
- partnerships involving a wider range of sectors – public, private and voluntary
- partnerships which co-ordinate multiple partnerships, such as LSPs.

In such circumstances the big debate of the late 1990s about the 'Berlin Wall' between the NHS and social care services – and by inference the care trust debate – seems less significant. By 2002, more than 40% of social services departments in England were combined with other services, local government was tackling its own cabinet/mayoral reorganisation and work was underway with a new range of partners such as Sure Start and Connexions. All of this calls for the development of new working relationships within local government. As a recent review of partnerships by the King's Fund has noted (Banks, 2002, para 7.5):

> There are concerns that new boundaries are being created, particularly where structural arrangements are set up.

Human resources capacity

PCTs already face a huge HR agenda which will leave little scope for taking on a parallel agenda for social care – indeed they will find it difficult to deliver upon their own concerns. Guidance outlines the scale of the challenge:

> Care trusts will be formed by bringing together staff from the NHS and the local council. While most staff are likely to transfer to the new

organisation under arrangements which transfer their terms and conditions of service (TUPE), secondments will also be possible, as will new appointments when new posts are created.

(DoH, 2001a, p 8)

None of this will be achieved without difficulty. Several issues can be identified.

- **TUPE:** Staff will have their old terms and conditions of service protected under either a transfer order or the Transfer of Undertakings (Protection of Employment) Regulations, but care trusts will want to move towards common terms and conditions for all staff. Existing PCTs have found variations not only in pay for staff doing the same or similar jobs, but also in fringe benefits such as annual leave, and it remains unclear whether local authority staff transferring to a care trust can remain in the local government pension scheme.
- **Legislative observance:** A range of potential legal problems will need to be recognised and addressed including: reconciliation of different disciplinary proceedings, implementing equal opportunities – an issue likely to be more focused for social services, implementing 'whistle blowing' and human rights legislation.
- **HR support to GPs:** PCTs have been given the job of providing HR support to GPs, but have no powers other than persuasion and control over some discretionary funds. The varied record of GPs as employers will be a difficult task to address.
- **Challenges to professional constituencies:** Integrating the community and practice nursing workforces will be a key task for PCTs – in the Tracker Survey, 77% of PCGs planning to become PCTs mentioned this as one of the three most important reasons for wanting trust status (Wilkin *et al.*, 2001). The formation of fully integrated nursing teams with common management and contracts remains a challenge to be met.

PCTs typically have no real HR infrastructure to deliver on this agenda. Few of them are going to be big enough to justify a full HR department and will need to buy in support from an acute or community trust or develop a consortium with other PCTs. In the meantime 80% of the one million strong social care workforce have no formal qualifications or training for the job and achievement on the national quality standard for staff development – Investors in People – is hampered by lack of resources. The idea that the HR agenda for social care can be tacked on to this in a care trust is therefore to be treated with caution. Trades unions have been understandably alarmed – UNISON members, for example, have called on their leaders to promote alternative mechanisms to care trusts that do not require members to transfer out of local authority employment.

The impact of organisational upheaval

The organisational turbulence that has already occurred in the NHS, combined with the prospect of even further radical change, makes prosecution of the joint agenda difficult. PCTs face a big challenge in taking over much of the role previously performed by health authorities, as the latter transmogrify into StHAs (DoH, 2001b). They will keep their current roles, but also be responsible for the provision of mental health services, for managing dentistry, optometry and pharmacy, as well as having responsibility for key links with local government. Some may have been reasonably well prepared for this eventuality by their 'old' health authorities, but most have not. The second Tracker Survey, for example, showed only 15% of PCG/T chief officers reporting their health authority to be actively supporting them – a drop of 2% on the previous year (Wilkin *et al.*, 2001).

The prospect of even more structural change through care trusts will only further detract from a focus upon these challenges. A survey of NHS chief executives on reactions to *Shifting the Balance of Power within the NHS* (Walshe and Smith, 2001) certainly suggests little appetite on the part of NHS managers for further reorganisation. The authors report:

- 75% felt that reorganisation would delay the delivery of *The NHS Plan* over the coming year, with a quarter saying the delay would be 'severe'
- 55% expressed negative views about the reorganisation
- on average chief executives were spending 25% of their time implementing the reforms
- almost half were concerned about PCTs' abilities to cope with an enlarged set of responsibilities.

These findings are reflected in the formal responses to *Shifting the Balance of Power within the NHS: securing delivery*. The follow-up document, *Shifting the Balance of Power: the next steps* (DoH, 2002) notes that over 400 responses were received, with four prominent concerns being expressed:

- the pace of change and speed of movement
- the capacity of PCTs to take on their role fully from April 2002
- the disruption the changes may cause
- the ability of health authorities/StHAs to hold the programme together while they are reorganising.

Even without the next step towards care trusts, this upheaval in the NHS has impacted upon the social care agenda and the prospects for partnership between the NHS and social care.

Poor partnership record of PCTs

Although the notion of a care trust is that PCTs and local councils can further build upon a good record of joint working, there is little evidence to suggest that partnership with social services or the local authority has been much of a priority for PCTs. An initial problem is the lack of co-terminosity between local authority and PCT boundaries. The government's line is half-hearted in this respect, expressing little more than a wish to move towards the alignment of boundaries 'where it is sensible to do so' (NHS Executive, 1999). The latest Tracker Survey (Wilkin *et al.*, 2001) reports 'extensive differences' in the geographic boundaries of PCG/Ts and local authorities (para 10.8) – a quarter of PCG/Ts were found to cover patients in local authorities not represented on the PCG/T board. Moreover, 29% of social services representatives said their department's budgets were not devolved or aligned with the PCG/Ts boundaries, and decisions about operational and service delivery were not aligned for 39% of PCG/Ts. Social services seem keen to improve this situation. The survey found almost two-thirds were planning changes in the coming year in some aspect of their operations in order to improve alignment with PCG/Ts, but these efforts did not appear to be reciprocated. In only 20% of PCG/Ts did the desire to align boundaries or achieve better co-ordination with local authority services feature as a reason for planned mergers or moves to trust status.

This relative disinterest in co-terminosity is further reflected in the low engagement of social services representatives in the machinery of PCG/T governance. Again, the Tracker Survey reveals that in 2000, even fewer social services representatives held office on the PCG/T board than in 1999 – only two were vice-chairs and nine chairs of sub-committees or working groups. Glendinning *et al.* (2001, p 422) conclude that:

> The statutory requirement for PCG boards to include a representative from the local social services department is, in many instances, only a partial gesture towards the development of inter-agency relationships ... (their) full participation was restricted by their perceived lack of influence compared to other categories of board members.

The Health Act flexibilities deserve a chance

Even with good local disposition towards partnership working, it is asking too much of too many PCTs to expect them to take the further step to care trust status. But the more fundamental issue is whether such a move is wise or necessary. Care trusts and section 31 partnership arrangements are both means to the same end – more integrated service delivery; the question is, which is most likely to fulfil that purpose? Localities wishing to apply for care trust status are required to complete a self-audit tool to judge their readiness to make the transition. One of the requirements is that local partners should have a good record of joint working and be able to justify a proposal for a care trust rather than use of the Health Act flexibilities (DoH, 2001c). The case for care trust status therefore becomes one of whether such a position offers added value over and above the benefits arising from good partnership working and effective use of section 31. It is not clear that this case can be strongly made.

Conclusion: networks not structures?

Initial guidance on the development of care trusts (DoH, 2001a) was honest enough to confess that 'care trusts alone cannot solve the difficult issues that arise when there are complex services to co-ordinate'. The message of this chapter is that it is not clear whether care trusts constitute *any* sort of an answer to the causes of fragmented service delivery. Paradoxically, the interest in an 'Old Labour' solution – structures – has re-appeared at a time when there is widespread recognition that partnership working increasingly has to respond to 'wicked issues' that transcend any restructuring solution. This new requirement can be distinguished from the issues that can be addressed by 'old partnerships'. 'Old partnerships' are typified by the arrangements which developed for resettlement from long-stay hospitals, especially in the case of learning difficulties. Whilst it is important to avoid regarding contexts such as this as 'simple', there nevertheless tend to be elements in place which make a successful outcome more likely. Such features are similar to the characteristics of what Challis *et al.* (1988) have described as 'planned bargaining':

- partnerships come together with the intention of delivering pre-set common objectives
- there is confidence that the objectives are the right ones, based upon experience of what works
- the focus is the resolution of existing problems rather than the anticipation of future ones
- partnership working is relatively small scale and ad hoc, rather than part of a broader partnership design.

Partnerships of this type will continue to have an important role to play, but increasingly it will be necessary to participate in new partnerships related to different sorts of issues. The conceptual underpinning of the notion of 'new partnerships' has two elements. First the shift from government to governance. Governance is a broader term than government, with services provided by any permutation of the statutory, private and voluntary sectors. The complexity arising out of this functional differentiation of the state makes inter-agency linkages a defining characteristic of service delivery. Rhodes (1997) goes on to define governance as 'self-organising inter-organisational networks' characterised by interdependence between agencies, continuing interactions between partners arising from the need to exchange resources and negotiate shared purposes, and some degree of autonomy from the state, which can only indirectly and imperfectly steer networks.

The second feature is the growing focus upon 'wicked issues'. For Clarke and Stewart (1997) these issues constitute those policy matters that are particularly difficult to resolve because:

- the problem itself is hard to define
- the causal chains are difficult (if not impossible) to unravel
- complex interdependencies are involved.

In this context, organisational structures and boundaries, and any reshuffling of them as with care trusts, become a secondary matter. In so far as there is a 'system' it refers to something that assembles itself around a shared purpose and the key issue is 'what is the right mix of people for that purpose and how do their voices get heard?' (Pratt *et al.*, 1999). New Labour has, at least in part, turned its back on markets, but seems unable to decide between hierarchy and network as its guiding principle. Wicked issues are best suited to a network approach nested in the partnership imperative; they are ill-suited to a fixation with structural change through care trusts.

There is no simple way to 'build networks'. Network structures are characterised by a decentralised negotiating style which trades off control for agreement. As Rhodes (1999, p 12) comments, 'this means agreeing with the objectives of others, not just persuading them that you were right all along, or resorting to sanctions when they disagree'. This in turn implies a localised nature, often leading to 'dense' transactions – the network will be organised around shared meaning and members will organise locally in tune with the network. Spatial constraint will be a further dimension here, since networks will operate in environments that are naturally bounded or artificially created.

Such a scenario assumes the voluntary creation of networks – the normal expectation – but the relationship between the emergence of local networks and the role of an executive steering body is complex. Although networks 'work' where they self-organise around a co-created and meaningful purpose, an executive authority also has a role to play, and it is here, rather than in the promotion of care trusts, that the government needs to be putting its effort. The first role is to ensure an environment that encourages networks, and to develop new processes for policy formation and implementation that make the most of the potential of networks – the *enabling role*. A central department can, for example, provide the policy framework and guidance, prod the network into action by systematic review and scrutiny, and mobilise resources and skills across sectors.

A second role is where the state does indeed attempt to create and drive networks – the *implementation role*. In England, a range of local networks around 'zones' for education, employment and health have been centrally driven. Far from being voluntary or autonomous, these kinds of networks are used by government as a means of implementing policy at the local level. Incentives in the form of additional money are provided to generate interest in networks as a means of gathering together stakeholders in new forms of inter-agency and cross-sectoral working. These networks differ from the voluntary, autonomous and independent networks described by Rhodes. The extent of their autonomy is undermined by a closeness to central government initiatives in the competition for resources; their voluntary access and membership is similarly undermined where, in order to gain advantage, it becomes impossible to stay outside of the network.

The network is likely to be time-limited to realising its own goals, with clear entry and exit criteria established, but this sort of precision has to be balanced against the relative fluidity of the relationships. Because networks are likely to *evolve*, the precise nature of the relationships between the elements of the network is likely to be ambiguous and there will have to be a high tolerance for ambiguity and uncertainty. Jackson and Stainsby (2000, p 13) argue that since networks are, by nature, 'a myriad of connections and relationships', then they will 'evolve in a kaleidoscopic fashion'. Linear managerial thinking, starting with strategy and moving to implementation and review, is too simplistic for this mode of governance.

All in all, the government has basically got it wrong when it comes to care trusts and handled it badly. Far better to identify the problems and review ways of addressing them effectively, than push for an unwarranted and potentially disastrous structural reorganisation.

References

Bamford T (2001) *Commissioning and Purchasing.* Routledge and Community Care, London.

Banks P (2002) *Partnerships Under Pressure.* King's Fund, London.

Challis L, Fuller S, Henwood M *et al.* (1988) *Joint Approaches to Social Policy: rationality and practice.* Cambridge University Press, Cambridge.

Clarke M and Stewart J (1997) *Handling the Wicked Issues: a challenge for government.* Institute of Local Government Studies, University of Birmingham, Birmingham.

Department of Health (2000) *The NHS Plan: a plan for investment, a plan for reform.* TSO, London.

Department of Health (2001a) *Care Trusts: emerging framework.* DoH, London.

Department of Health (2001b) *Shifting the Balance of Power within the NHS: securing delivery.* DoH, London.

Department of Health (2001c) *Care Trust Application, Consultation, Assessment and Establishment Processes.* DoH, London.

Department of Health (2002) *Shifting the Balance of Power: the next steps.* DoH, London.

Glendinning C, Abbott S and Coleman A (2001) Bridging the gap: new relationships between primary care groups and local authorities. *Social Policy and Administration.* **35**(4): 411–25.

Health Select Committee (1998) *The Relationship between Health and Social Services: volume 1.* TSO, London.

Henwood M (2001) *The Health and Social Care Interface: from partnership to integration?* Paper to Health and Social Care Conference in Britain and Europe Conference, London School of Economics, 10 January 2002, London.

Hudson B (2002a) Ten reasons not to trust care trusts. *Managing Community Care.* **10**(2): 3–11.

Hudson B (2002b) Integrated care and structural change in England: the case of care trusts. *Policy Studies.* **23**(2): 77–95.

Hudson B, Young R, Hardy B *et al.* (2001) *National Evaluation of Notifications for Use of the section 31 Partnership Flexibilities of the Health Act 1999: second interim report.* Nuffield Institute for Health/National Primary Care Research and Development Centre, Leeds/Manchester.

Jackson PM and Stainsby L (2000) Managing public sector networked organisations. *Public Money and Management.* January–March: 11–16.

National Health Service Executive (1999) *Establishing Primary Care Groups.* Health Service Circular 1998/065.

Peck E, Towell D and Gulliver P (2001) The meanings of 'culture' in health and social care: a case study of the combined trust in Somerset. *J Interprofessional Care.* **15**(4): 319–27.

Platt D (2001) *Modern Social Services: a commitment to deliver – the 10th Annual Report of the Chief Inspector of Social Services, Social Services Inspectorate.* DoH, London.

Pratt J, Gordon P and Plamping D (1999) *Whole Systems Working: putting theory into practice in organisations*. King's Fund, London.

Rhodes RAW (1997) *Understanding Governance: policy networks, governance, reflexivity and accountability*. Open University Press, Buckinghamshire.

Rhodes RAW (1999) *The Governance Narrative: key findings and lessons from the ESRC's Whitehall programme*. Economic and Social Research Council, London.

Royal Commission on Long Term Care (1999) *With Respect to Old Age: long term care – rights and responsibilities*. TSO, London.

Social Services Inspectorate (2000) *Review of Care in the Community*. Department of Health, Social Services and Public Safety, Belfast.

Walshe K and Smith J (2001) Cause and effect. *Health Service J*. 11 October: 20–1.

Wilkin D, Gillam S and Coleman A (2001) *The National Tracker Survey of Primary Care Groups and Trusts 2000/2001: modernising the NHS*. King's Fund/National Primary Care Research and Development Centre, London/Manchester.

CHAPTER 8

The Northumberland experience

Lucy O'Leary

Background

Northumberland is the most northerly county in England, stretching from the banks of the Tyne northwards to the Scottish border, and from the North Sea coast westwards to the Pennines. In all, it covers an area of approximately 2000 square miles. With a population of around 312 000, it is the least densely populated county of England. The county has two-tier local government with a county council responsible for delivery of social services and six district councils providing a range of local services including housing. Until April 2002, the area was served by a single health authority co-terminous with the county council and four PCGs (covering North, West and Central Northumberland and Blyth Valley in the south-east of the county). There are 54 GP practices.

Northumberland suffers from extremes of poverty. Urban populations, such as those in the south-east of the county, have some of the lowest average incomes in the country. As well as a low average, some districts also exhibit very significant inequalities of income. The European Commission recognises that north-east England has been particularly affected by economic decline, with unemployment a major problem. Rural isolation is highlighted by the fact that England's most deprived ward, taking into account access to services, lies in North Northumberland. Getting services to people who need them most when they live in isolated and dispersed communities is a major challenge for all local agencies. The full impact of the foot and mouth crisis of 2001 has yet to be fully assessed at the time of writing, but it has had a significant effect on the rural economy and the health of people living in rural communities.

In health terms, the population of Northumberland fares considerably less well than the England and Wales average. The inequalities evident in health determinants such as employment, income, housing and access to services are, unsurprisingly, reflected in the wide contrasts in health within the county. The health issues causing the most significant demand for services are the same as in the rest of the UK: heart disease and stroke, cancer, mental health problems and the needs of the growing older population.

Joint working in Northumberland – a brief history

There is a strong track record of partnership working between Northumberland agencies aimed at tackling health problems in their widest sense. This perhaps reflects both a culture of self-sufficiency and resourcefulness, and recognition of the role of the wider public sector in determining health and well-being gained from the experience of the economic decline of the 1970s and 1980s. This recognition has resulted in the formation of inclusive partnerships to address Northumberland's needs, including health inequalities and social deprivation. The Northumberland Strategic Partnership was formed in 1997 to provide a county-wide framework for tackling these issues and it now works alongside the LSPs led by the six district councils. In each of these partnership initiatives, improved health and well-being are recognised as an objective of community development and regeneration. Northumberland was one of the first wave of HAZs in 1999 and the Northumberland HAZ was founded on the need for strong links across the local economy to tackle the determinants of ill health and to reduce health inequalities.

The community care reforms of the early 1990s provided the catalyst for new thinking by the county council and local NHS organisations about service models and the potential advantages of working together to achieve shared service goals. This resulted in a range of services developed and provided jointly from 1993 onwards. These include integrated care management teams for people with mental health needs, people with a learning disability and younger people with a physical impairment. These teams bring together social workers and health professionals (most often nurses and occupational therapists) into a single team, with any of these professionals able to provide the care management function for service users. These teams were, until April 2002, managed within social services, with the NHS team members seconded in and with professional supervision provided in parallel to line management of the teams.

In 1994, a further development created a single budget for care management, formed by the transfer of funding from the health authority to the county council. Care management teams thus had access to a single pooled budget for the purchase of services for clients. Equipment services were integrated with a single store and a single ordering and loan system, hosted by the local acute and community NHS trust. Other new services were developed by agencies on a project basis including, in 2000, four locality-based community rehabilitation teams providing intermediate care for older people following a stroke. Wherever possible, social care services and health services have been co-located, often within primary care premises (although given the dispersed population in the county and the scope offered by existing accommodation, this has not been possible everywhere). Care management teams have been organised on a patch basis covering a group of practices, providing a consistent access point for service users and professionals.

The development of these jointly provided services was balanced by a partnership approach to service planning and commissioning. During the 1990s, the Northumberland Policy Group provided the main forum for agencies to discuss strategies for improving health for local people, to develop the Northumberland

Health Improvement Programme and to agree on investment priorities. The policy group included senior representation from:

- Northumberland Health Authority
- Northumberland County Council (both Chief Executive and Director of Social Services being members of the group)
- the four Northumberland PCGs formed in April 1999
- Newcastle Hospitals NHS Trust (providing acute healthcare in Newcastle, especially tertiary services, for Northumberland residents)
- Northumberland Mental Health NHS Trust
- Northgate and Prudhoe NHS Trust (providing learning disability services)
- Northumbria Healthcare NHS Trust (providing acute and community health care in Northumberland and North Tyneside).

(In 2000 and following the publication of *The NHS Plan* (DoH, 2000), the policy group was re-established as the Northumberland Modernisation Board with the same partner organisations.)

The journey towards the care trust: from *The NHS Plan* to *Shifting the Balance of Power within the NHS*

By early 2000, debate had been taking place for some time within the Northumberland Strategic Partnership about how joint working and integration could continue to develop in Northumberland. This was based in part on a feeling that not enough was being done to build on the pioneering work of the 1990s and that there was a need to re-energise local partners to drive further forward with integration.

Work began on a whole systems review of health and social care services in the county, led by a group drawn from the Northumberland Policy Group and including the chief executives of the local NHS organisations, together with the Chief Executive of the County Council and the Director of Social Services. One objective of this work was to enable agreement to be reached on the number and configuration of PCTs for Northumberland. A number of options were explored with GPs, primary care staff, the PCGs, other stakeholders and the public. Agreement was reached in spring 2000 that the favoured option was a single PCT for Northumberland, provided that this was founded on four strong localities corresponding to the PCGs.

Shortly after this decision had been reached, *The NHS Plan* was published, launching the concept of a care trust as a means of integrating health and social care services in a single organisation. The Whole Systems Review Group was immediately interested in the potential benefits offered by the care trust idea, particularly by the model based on a PCT and including integration of both commissioning and provision. However, the absence of any detailed guidance or practical timetable for establishment at this early stage meant that the group did not feel able to make a formal expression of interest. In particular, it was felt that elected council members would need more information on care trust governance and the links between the care trust and the council in order to agree to an application.

The Whole Systems Review Group was reconvened in January 2001 as the Northumberland PCT/Care Trust Project Board, to oversee development work towards the changes to take place in April 2002. Discussions were held with the NHS Regional Office and the DoH on the emerging care trust model and the likely timescales for the first tranche.

A key point in this early work was the development of a Northumberland shared vision for health and social care, led by the project board with the involvement of a wide range of other stakeholders including the district councils and the community health council. The vision was that, in Northumberland, health and social care services should be:

- better organised
- easier to understand
- provided when and where they are needed.

This simply expressed vision of services provided the starting point for the development of the PCT and care trust model, and continues to be at the centre of the care trust's strategy.

A further driver for change at this point was the publication by the DoH, in spring 2001, of *Shifting the Balance of Power within the NHS: securing delivery* (DoH, 2001). Although this did not address the issue of care trust development, the proposed changes to NHS organisations were of direct relevance to the work being carried out in Northumberland in a number of ways.

1 The proposed new structures, with the replacement of the former Northumberland Health Authority by a new StHA with a larger catchment area, provided additional justification for the development of a single primary care organisation for the county, as opposed to a number of smaller organisations serving only part of Northumberland. This was widely seen as essential in order to protect the interests of Northumberland people and services within a new health authority area also including the Tyne and Wear conurbation (an area with very different demography, service models and development priorities).

2 The new role of the PCT as the lead NHS organisation in assessing need, planning and commissioning, and improving health was seen to support a 'maximal care trust' model with the transfer of all or most social care services from the county council. This would bring together health and social care services both in commissioning and in primary and community care provision, with maximum potential for co-ordination between the two arms of the overall service.

3 The timing of the organisational changes set out in *Shifting the Balance of Power within the NHS* meant that April 2002 was increasingly seen as the most logical starting date for the Northumberland Care Trust. There was a strong preference within the project board for as few phases of organisational change as possible and, if at all possible, a single point at which services and staff would come together in a new organisation. The formation of a PCT in April 2002, followed at some future date by a further change bringing in social care staff to create a care trust, was seen as likely to prolong the inevitable period of disruption for staff. It was also felt that, in a two-stage change process, social care would be

more likely to be seen as a 'junior partner' joining a healthcare organisation, rather than both sets of services coming together in a full partnership from the start. *Shifting the Balance of Power within the NHS*, with its proposals for the transfer of functions, and therefore staff, from the old health authority to the new PCT in April 2002, added further weight to this argument.

Despite the uncertainties in the system at this time, the group was keen to explore the care trust concept and the options for development with local stakeholders. An extensive programme of pre-consultation was arranged, wherever possible tapping into existing meetings held by staff and other stakeholders. The proposed change to a single Northumberland PCT in April 2002 was explained, as was the concept of a care trust, which could be developed as an alternative model with the same target date. In all, over 1700 people were involved in these meetings.

The pre-consultation stage revealed a considerable level of support amongst frontline health and social care staff for the concept of an integrated organisation, despite the lack of clarity about how and when it could happen. This is perhaps a reflection of the number of staff with direct experience of working in integrated services, or in teams located alongside colleagues from other organisations and professions. There were, inevitably, many questions about the impact such a change would have on individual services and employees, as well as some concerns (from both health and social care) that 'the other side' would be seen to have a higher priority in the new organisation, especially in terms of funding and investment. Other stakeholders from the voluntary and independent sectors, and the community health council, also expressed considerable interest in the idea of a care trust at this early stage. Overall, the feeling was that this was an interesting idea that appeared to provide an opportunity to take integration a stage further in Northumberland, if the nuts and bolts of achieving such a change could be effectively managed.

Consultations, decisions and application

By July 2001, the project board was confident that a proposal to establish a care trust would achieve support from front-line staff and local stakeholders. However, there was still no government guidance on governance and accountability and therefore it had not been possible to debate the issue formally within the county council nor to consult the wider Northumberland public. The *Shifting the Balance of Power within the NHS* timetable meant that formal consultation on establishing a PCT was now necessary and this went ahead from July to October 2001. The consultation proposal highlighted the care trust as a possible future option and consultees were asked to comment on the option of establishing a care trust at a future date, if it was not possible to do so in one step in April 2002. The PCT consultation resulted in overall support for the establishment of a county-wide organisation, with additional support expressed for the care trust option if achievable.

Almost as soon as the PCT consultation had begun, draft DoH guidance on care trust governance and accountability was issued, thus enabling the debate to be taken forward with elected members as well as the project board partners. It became clear that there was support for the concept within the council, and that the governance proposals provided the level of assurance required to go ahead to a public consultation. Both the decision to consult, and the subsequent decision to make an application, were approved both by the council executive and by a full meeting of the council.

The county council, the health authority and the NHS trusts were each asked to agree to a further period of consultation on a proposal to establish a PCT-based care trust, with April 2002 as the favoured start date. This consultation took place in November and December 2001.

During this time, work on the detail of the proposed care trust was continuing along many parallel lines. Work streams had been developed at an early stage, reporting into the project board via a larger project team, which had begun by considering both the PCT-only and the care trust options for April 2002. At this point, work on the care trust option was stepped up. Workstreams included:

- clinical and care governance
- commissioning
- communications
- finance
- governance
- HR and organisational development
- IM&T
- locality management
- non-clinical support services
- partnerships
- service provision.

Some fundamentals had been discussed and agreed by the project board at early stages. In particular, the question of whether children's services should transfer from the council to a care trust had been extensively debated. Although the shared vision applied equally to services for children and adults, it was agreed that the additional complexities of children's services, especially the wider partnerships with education and other services, meant that they should remain within the council's direct management for the present. (Subsequent government proposals for integrated children's trusts hosted by local authorities have made it unlikely that children's social services will be transferred to the care trust. Any further integration would be likely to be in the opposite direction, with the child health services now provided by the care trust transferred to a children's trust. However, at the time of writing there are no plans to establish a children's trust in Northumberland.)

The response to this second consultation was extremely positive, the most significant of a very small number of objections being the response received from UNISON in line with its national position on care trust development. In January 2002, therefore, the project board, the health authority and the county council agreed to the submission of a formal application to the Secretary of State for the establishment of Northumberland Care Trust on 1 April 2002. The application was approved and the care trust duly established in the first tranche. The main structures and service models on which the application was based are described in the sections which follow.

The care trust now: key themes and issues

Governance and accountability

Northumberland Care Trust has followed the standard model for care trust governance, with a number of local arrangements running in parallel which meet the particular needs of local people and stakeholder organisations. The Care Trust Board includes three elected county councillors as non-executive directors, nominated by the council. It was agreed that two of these posts should be taken by the council's majority party and one by the opposition. DoH governance guidelines for PCT-based care trusts provide for a GP and a nurse representative from the Professional Executive Committee (PEC) to serve on the Board. In Northumberland, one of the social worker members of the PEC has also been identified as a Board member. The Board consists of:

- a lay Chair
- four lay non-executive directors appointed by the NHS Appointments Commission (one from 2003 as a representative of the patients' forum)
- three county councillors nominated by the council
- the Chief Executive
- the Director of Finance
- the Director of Clinical and Care Governance
- the Director of Public Health
- the Director of Social Care and Planning
- the Chair of the PEC
- the GP representative from the PEC
- the nurse representative from the PEC
- the social worker representative from the PEC (co-opted)
- the four locality directors (co-opted).

The PEC itself has a wider membership than the standard model, to reflect the need for strong presence from the localities as well as from a range of professionals. (There is agreement on the formal voting membership of the PEC in line with the standard model). The full PEC membership consists of:

- the executive directors
- the locality directors
- four GPs (one from each locality)
- four nurses (one from each locality)
- four social workers (one from each locality)
- two other professionals (currently a physiotherapist and an occupational therapist)
- the mental health trust's locality director for Northumberland.

Both the Board and PEC have had to address the question of individual members' roles. For the Board, this is particularly relevant for the councillor members, who are nominated by the council but who are full non-executive directors with equal roles and responsibilities to the other non-executives. Thus, while they will clearly have particular expertise and experience of the services previously managed directly by the council, they are responsible as part of the corporate whole for the entire range of functions carried out by the Care Trust and are not acting purely as representatives of the council.

At the PEC, the issue is one of balancing the need for the main groups in the Care Trust's professional and clinical workforce to have a voice with the need to achieve an effective corporate team to lead on service strategy and modernisation. National governance guidelines place some limits on the way in which professionals can be selected for the PEC (so that, for example, nurse, doctors and social workers must all be represented). The added need, in Northumberland, for all four localities to have an equal say in the PEC has meant a complex set of criteria for the places available to professionals. It is also potentially in conflict with the care trust's ethos of integration and flexible working between professionals, and much early development work has focused on the respective roles of 'representative' (of one's profession, locality, etc.) and 'champion' (someone able to work across professional and other boundaries and to bring the views of a range of professionals to the PEC table).

Accountability routes are often perceived as particularly complex for a PCT-based care trust. However, in essence they differ little from the way in which the constituent parts of the organisation have been accountable in the past. As an NHS organisation, the Care Trust is accountable through the Board to the StHA and the Secretary of State. It also accounts to Northumberland County Council (for the delivery of healthcare services) through the relatively new mechanism of the council's Scrutiny Committee. In terms of social care, legal responsibility for the delivery of social services in Northumberland remains with the council's Director of Social Services. The difference is that, whereas before April 2002 the Director of Social Services had direct control of staff and resources used to deliver social care to adults, these have now, with a few exceptions discussed below, transferred to the Care Trust. The Director of Social Services thus manages the relationship with the Care Trust through the partnership agreement and the annual agreement on delegated services.

The partnership agreement forms the strategic basis for the transfer of services and resources from the county council to the Care Trust. It is a section 31 agreement under the Health Act 1999, covering the totality of the transferred functions rather than, as in previous use of Health Act flexibilities, specific individual services. While in some other areas this has been interpreted as a detailed legal document, the approach in Northumberland was:

> ... to set out clearly the undertakings given by each party and the intended basis of their relationship. It is the intention of the parties to operate the agreement in a spirit of mutual trust as partners. The mechanism envisaged for resolution of any disputes is arbitration ... rather than legal action.

This approach was accepted by all the partner organisations at an early stage of the development work, greatly assisting the process of drafting and finalising the agreement in the run-up to April 2002. Since then, it has been used as a practical tool for managing the relationship between the council and the Care Trust.

Finance

The total budget for the Care Trust in 2002/03 is approximately £375 million. Of this, around £87m has been transferred to the Care Trust from the county council. This includes the previously developed pooled budget for care management, totalling £74m, with £8m of this representing healthcare funding from the Care Trust. The partnership agreement states that there is a clear intention to develop a fully pooled budget in the long term. However, the need to ensure budget stability in the early stages and to provide reassurance to the partners led to an agreement that funding received from the council would initially be ring-fenced within the overall Care Trust budget. Any extensions to the existing pooled budget arrangements require specific agreement from the council.

Service provision

The 'maximal care trust' ideal discussed above has been translated into an organisation providing a wide range of services. The original PCT proposal included the transfer of all community-based NHS health services (except adult mental health) from their existing trusts to the new organisation. The process of negotiation during the development period led to some services remaining within the original trusts, although some (such as the six community hospitals in Northumberland, currently part of Northumbria Healthcare NHS Trust) remain as subjects for future discussion and potential future transfer. However, the Care Trust's health service portfolio is extensive including, for example, child health, occupational therapy, wheelchair services, podiatry and speech and language therapy.

Community based mental health services for adults were excluded from the proposal because of pre-existing plans to provide an integrated health and social care service for adults of working age with mental health needs within the local mental health NHS trust. This meant that, whereas other care management services were transferred to the Care Trust, social care staff working in integrated care management teams for adults with mental health needs transferred to the Mental Health Trust. The links between the services provided by the two organisations are maintained through the PEC (the Mental Health Trust's locality manager is a member), the Northumberland Modernisation Board, locality management arrangements and the emerging mental health carestream, which includes the existing work on the mental health NSF.

The Care Trust's creation has totally transformed the model of provision for adult social care services. Services transferred to the Care Trust include the social care elements of:

- care management teams for older people (including teams for older people with mental health needs) and people with learning disabilities or physical disabilities
- integrated rehabilitation teams
- support functions for adult social services.

The council's 'provider services' – home care, residential homes, day care centres and so on – have not been transferred, although the Care Trust now manages these on behalf of the council under an agreement running in parallel with the partnership agreement. In many cases, there are plans for future changes in these services, such as reprovision of residential care by the independent sector or the development of 'social firms' for employment services, and for this reason it was felt that disruption could be minimised by excluding them from the initial stage of transfer. However, the Care Trust and the council continues to look at all the options for these services and it is possible that some may eventually transfer into the Care Trust.

The fundamental basis of all services provided by the Care Trust is that they will be managed within a single structure for health and social care, within localities wherever possible. This means that locality directors have a crucial role as the heads of the local 'delivery arms' of the organisation. The task of building this new management structure is still, at the time of writing, work in progress – an alternative approach to areas which have chosen to develop an integrated management structure before, or instead of, applying for care trust status.

Service planning and commissioning

The Care Trust's locality structure provides a strong basis for local needs assessment and prioritisation. Localities lead on commissioning primary, community and intermediate health and social care for their own area, working together as necessary with provider organisations (and in this respect it is important to note the high level of personal medical services (PMS) pilots in Northumberland – almost 75% – with one locality totally covered by a single PMS organisation). They then work together with the Care Trust's core planning and commissioning functions to commission secondary, tertiary and specialised services on a county-wide basis.

However, the Care Trust is also committed to developing a carestream approach to commissioning, in which care needs, service provision and modernisation are addressed across the whole system of health and social care for the big issues affecting local people: conditions like coronary heart disease, cancer or mental health, and priority groups like children, older people and those with a learning disability, to take some examples. The carestream approach challenges traditional commissioning and planning structures, and requires very effective leadership, networking and communication skills. Matching this approach with locality-based knowledge and experience, and with the expectations of a range of stakeholders from service users and carers to NHS trusts, the independent sector and professional groups, is possibly the most significant task for the Care Trust in its first years. Much of the organisational development required is around the development of the carestream approach and its implications for staff and stakeholders.

Primary care

As a PCT-based Care Trust, Northumberland is tackling the full range of issues, common to all PCTs, relating to primary care development. The majority of practices work within a PMS contract, and two localities have a single PMS organisation covering all or virtually all practices. The establishment of the Care Trust has reinforced the importance of integration and joint working at practice level (and there are many long-standing local examples of this) and appropriate objectives are being built into contractual arrangements with both PMS and GMS practices.

Implementation of GP appraisal is a major project for all PCTs. The approach in Northumberland has been to work on a common approach for all staff groups including those in primary healthcare teams (whether employed by the practice or by the Care Trust). The Care Trust is committed to establishing team-based appraisal working with delivery teams including those in primary care. This raises questions of who should be the appraiser in a multi-disciplinary team context and on the links between appraisal and other dimensions of clinical governance tackling specific professional/clinical challenges.

A new workforce

By the end of 2002, the Care Trust employed directly approximately 1200 staff, of which around 25% had previously been employed by the county council, 10% by the health authority or a PCG, and 65% by one of the NHS trusts. A further 5000 staff are employed as part of the Care Trust 'family': either by a primary care practice or in the council provider services managed by the Care Trust.

Clearly, the employment and workforce issues facing the Care Trust go beyond the practicalities of transferring social care staff to the NHS. In fact, although issues such as pensions and continuity of service were very important in the run-up to April 2002, the key priorities for the organisation now are just as much about achieving effective staff involvement and good, consistent two-way communications as in the essentials of joint policies, procedures and in moving towards harmonisation of terms and conditions.

The changes inherent in moving to an integrated management structure and a carestream approach to planning and delivery are significant for all groups of staff. Traditional, hierarchical structures will not be able to meet the need for flexible working across professional, carestream or organisational boundaries. The Care Trust is committed to a new way of working in which arrangements for line management and professional supervision sit alongside the need for flexible team-working and innovation. This continues to require extensive work with unions and with staff as a whole to share the new vision, understand and respond to staff concerns, and ensure that people feel they have a voice in the new organisation.

The early lessons

As will be clear from the comments above, the Care Trust is still (in January 2003) an emerging entity, full of uncertainty and grappling with a host of changes and challenges for the future. Yet the enthusiasm with which staff and partner organisations entered into the process of developing the new organisation is still there: frustrated by the inevitable delays in being able to make changes on the ground, perhaps, but committed to doing things differently and moving towards the vision of health and social care services that are better organised, easier to understand and provided when and where they are needed.

It is absolutely certain that support for, and commitment to, a care trust would have been impossible to secure had it not been for the long history of effective partnership working in the county, providing people at all levels from top management to front-line and support staff with confidence in the potential benefits, assurance that the inevitable risks of further integration could be managed intelligently and experience of working alongside colleagues from a range of backgrounds.

What is less easy to demonstrate is the benefit of a care trust, as opposed to any other form of partnership working, to local people in Northumberland. It is, of course, true that all the changes in service provision and commissioning planned by the Care Trust could be achieved in another area through use of Health Act flexibilities or other local arrangements. How any of the expected changes are experienced by local people is yet to be assessed and there are no easy ways of identifying what improvements are due to 'care trustness' and what to better working which would have taken place anyway. Clearly, this problem of analysing the effectiveness of any given organisational model is not peculiar to Northumberland.

Perhaps, in the end, the decision in Northumberland to take the care trust step is a reflection of a desire to create something new that could re-energise existing partnership working and take it onto a new level, by developing a new way of doing things outside the boundaries of all the existing organisations. It also reflects a desire to bring people together in this new organisation as early as possible, enabling them to work together to forge a new shared identity from the inside, rather than work on joint structures followed by a change in governance and organisational form. The challenge now is to live up to expectations by delivering this new shared identity, with the acknowledged risk that the Care Trust will be seen as less innovative and different to what was envisaged (and promised) before April 2002.

Ultimately, the care trust route will not be for everyone. But in Northumberland there is a belief that it is the next logical step on the road to achieving the shared vision: that it can be a sustainable organisation with a 'can-do' approach and an effective champion for the needs of Northumberland people.

References

Department of Health (2000) *The NHS Plan: a plan for investment, a plan for reform.* TSO, London.

Department of Health (2001) *Shifting the Balance of Power within the NHS: securing delivery.* DoH, London.

CHAPTER 9

The Sandwell experience

Lotta Macfarlane

Traditionally, Sandwell has had a national reputation for its successful partnership working, particularly between health and social services (known locally as Social Inclusion and Health). Against this background, it is perhaps unsurprising that key players within the local economy would look to using a care trust model to deliver plans for integrated mental health services. From April 2003, the existing Black Country Mental Health NHS Trust (BCMHT) was redesignated as Sandwell Mental Health NHS and Social Care Trust, with responsibility for the delivery of:

- all health service functions currently within the remit of BCMHT (including adult mental health, old age psychiatry, children and adolescent mental health and specialised learning disability services)
- all adult mental health social care services.

As the new Care Trust goes live, therefore, the time seems right to contribute this chapter, based on our experiences of partnership working, the barriers we have faced and the lessons we have learnt.

Sandwell: background and context

Sandwell is located in the heart of the Black Country in the West Midlands. Instead of being based on a single town or city, the local authority consists of a cluster of distinctive neighbourhoods that have a strong cultural history of tradition and sense of community. As a metropolitan borough, Sandwell is situated to the west of Birmingham, covering an area of approximately 33 square miles, with a population of 282 900, occupying the main towns of Oldbury, Smethwick, Rowley Regis, Tipton, Wednesbury and West Bromwich. Overall, there is a robust and active local community, with a rich cultural mix (approximately 16% of local people are from a minority ethnic community).

Despite its active community, Sandwell has a high level of deprivation with low educational levels, high unemployment and poor housing. This results in higher numbers of vulnerable people living in the community who use mental health and substance misuse services. Data suggest that, on any given day, as many as 5000 Sandwell residents receive care from the BCMHT (BCMHT, 2002). In addition, primary care surveys have shown that at least 26% of the population consult their family GP each year with a mental health problem. As a result, the need to develop integrated and co-ordinated planning and service delivery that is responsive to service users and their carers is paramount.

In Sandwell, local agencies have a long history of working together. This includes partners from the statutory, voluntary and private sectors, as well as, more recently, service users and carers. A health partnership was created in 1996, within the civic partnership thematic structure, whose remit was to achieve greater integration of health and social care across Sandwell. This resulted in a commitment to developing new structures that would:

- enhance care to patients
- further develop the efficiencies and effectiveness conferred by 'single' partnership arrangements
- achieve a balance between 'central' borough-wide planning and delivery and increased sensitivity to local needs and aspirations
- achieve a significantly increased focus on investment in primary and community services
- maximise money spent on patient care and organisational development rather than the cost of sustaining independent and potentially competing board structures
- always consider the impact of change on all constituent partners.

This drive and commitment to make a real difference in the ways that health and social care services are commissioned and provided locally has, over a period of time, led to a range of shared initiatives such as:

- the establishment of joint community mental health teams with joint resource management
- single access criteria for continuing care
- dual access budgets for health and social care
- joint home loans equipment organisation
- membership of the Executive Director of Social Services on the previous Sandwell Health Authority Board
- investment in partnership development infrastructure through HAZ status
- joint general manager posts for adult mental health services
- strategic/commissioning managers for older people's services, adult mental health, learning disabilities and children's services
- health partnership co-ordinating group
- HAZ programme steering group
- healthy living networks.

Particularly significant for this chapter was the creation in 2001 of a learning disability partnership board and, in 2002, of a mental health partnership board using the Health Act 1999 flexibilities. Using lead commissioning and pooled budget arrangements, these partnership bodies now commission all learning disability and mental health services in Sandwell.

Mental health services

Sandwell traditionally had no history of providing its own mental health services and throughout the 1980s experienced a very low level of local provision, with health services provided at All Saints Hospital in Birmingham. Then in the early 1990s, with the advent of the Mental Illness Specific Grant, the opportunity was seized to undertake joint work in planning and setting up CMHTs. In many ways, this formed the initial impetus for partnership working within mental health services in the borough and the creation of the CMHTs was to act as the cornerstone for new services. Four teams were established, resourced jointly by health and social care and managed on a 50:50 basis. Early development led to a management structure that was responsible for resource management across agencies, in addition to professional supervision and accountability. This pattern of trust and joint working has extended to all aspects of the teams' functioning including community care budget responsibility.

Since 1999, further integration has been driven by the need to deliver the NSF for Mental Health (DoH, 1999), calling for new types of mental health services and moving away from generic CMHTs towards more specialised teams. It was against this background that local partners began to consider ways of re-organising local provision with a particular emphasis on:

- developing more integrated mental health services
- ensuring that new specialist mental health teams did not fragment existing provision
- supporting the provision of local services to Sandwell residents.

However, consequential to the changes taking place within the local health economy as a result of *Shifting the Balance of Power within the NHS* (DoH, 2001a), changes in personnel resulted in a temporary disengagement by the health authority and a sudden emerging vulnerability of essential joint planning for mental health services. With health taking the strategic lead on national priorities through the NSF, it was essential to ensure stability and engage key leaders in early discussions to consider plans for future services.

Thus, when the concept of a care trust was first suggested by the DoH, local partners in Sandwell were already thinking along these lines and had to some extent, anticipated national policy developments.

The experience of having established a learning disability partnership board to commission services contributed to the decision to consider a similar arrangement for mental health services and the emphasis turned towards finding ways to further integrate local service provision.

Exploring options for the future

In autumn 2001, senior directors and managers from health and social care set up a project board to consider future options for service configuration and to ensure that all relevant stakeholders were involved throughout the process. To support this, a project team and a number of specific sub-groups (including HR, finance and corporate governance) were established. Between October 2001 and February

2002, a series of meetings and seminars were undertaken to share ideas and discuss with staff, users, carers and other stakeholders the potential for integrating
services for people with learning disabilities and for people with mental health
problems. Due to their complexity, it was decided that further independent consideration should be given to child and adolescent mental health and old age
psychiatry (and these issues are still being addressed at the time of writing). The
core issues that emerged from these discussions included:

- a strong wish from service users and carers for learning disability and mental
  health services to be provided from separate organisations rather than within a
  single organisation as they had previously experienced under BCMHT
- no good reason for mental health and learning disability services to take the
  same route
- a recognition that further development would be required by children's and old
  age mental health services before integration into a provider organisation could
  be recommended
- substance misuse services should be integrated into a single provider
- concern of staff about transferring employment and losing pension rights
- opposition from UNISON to the concept of a care trust
- concern from the local authority that its responsibility and accountability would
  be diminished within a care trust.

These discussions led to the development of a list of benefit criteria, grouped
under service and organisational requirements, against which service models
could be judged (*see* Table 9.1).

At the same time, a potential 14 models for future service configuration were
identified including a range of both commissioning and provider functions. It was
at this stage that a workshop was organised with carer and user representatives,
staff representatives and staff and managers from health and social care to
undertake an option appraisal using the previously agreed benefit criteria. The
models were judged against the criteria that had been individually weighted and
the final score resulted in seven ranked options (*see* Table 9.2).

The option evaluation concluded that the first three options were clearly ahead
of the others. These options were subsequently considered and combined appropriately to form the proposals that were put forward as part of the formal consultation process undertaken within Sandwell between 1 August and 31 October
2002. In particular, partner agencies recommended the creation of a single employer
organisation (a care trust for mental health, led by the health service) and an
integrated community service for people with learning disabilities (led by the
local authority). In both service areas, staff would transfer employment to the
relevant organisation (except for approved social workers, who would have to
remain seconded under current mental health legislation).

The rationale used by partner agencies in recommending this option as the
preferred choice included the following points.

- Mental health and learning disability services would have clear and separate
  identities. A local authority lead for learning disability services was seen as
  particularly important in light of the emphasis of *Valuing People* (DoH, 2001b)
  on wider services such as education, leisure and housing.

Table 9.1   Criteria for evaluating service proposals

Formal criteria	Explanations
Service issues	
1 Uses a whole systems approach.	Helps us to help service users by giving them exactly what they need at the time they need it. For example, some people feel depressed and need short-term help; others suffer for a long time and when feeling better need help to get back into work. This approach means we have thought of all that service users may need and how we fit it together.
2 Promotes partnership working to include involving users and carers at all levels from individual care to service planning and monitoring.	Helps us to see what service users and carers need through their eyes. An example of this would be finding out from the service user what would help them most, whether it is housing, counselling or help in a crisis, and working together to provide it.
3 Enables fair, fast, timely access to consistent local services 24 hours per day.	Helps all those who need a service to get that service quickly – no matter where they live or who they are.
4 Enables access to specialist services.	Helps those who need a service for a particular need/condition to get that service.
5 The public face of the organisation gives a focus on mental health and learning disability services and a voice to service users (thereby commanding service user and carer confidence).	Makes sure that we can invest in services that are needed and can listen and respond to service users.
Organisational issues	
6 Promotes policy orientation and accountability to the Secretary of State for Health.	Makes sure we give local people the services they have a right to receive (i.e. help when suffering distress).
7 Promotes policy orientation and accountability to the local authority.	Makes sure we give local people the services they have a right to receive (i.e. help sorting out housing and family worries).
8 Commands staff confidence and facilitates recruitment and retention.	Helps staff to have value and pride in the service.
9 Is flexible and enables further change.	Is able to change easily over time to make a better service.
10 Is affordable, sustainable and value for money.	Is something we can afford to do now and have enough money to keep running in the future.
11 Level of complexity makes the option less able to achieve all of the criteria.	Is too difficult to organise to meet the needs of the service.

Table 9.2 Service options

Rank	Model
1	Sandwell Mental Health Care Trust
2	Integrated Sandwell Care Trust
3	Health Act 1999 flexibilities
4	Mental Health PCT model
5	Integrated Sandwell local authority model
6	Sandwell & Birmingham Mental Health Care Trust
7	Integrated Sandwell PCT model

- A mental health care trust would prevent the new services introduced under the NSF for Mental Health from fragmenting local provision and give an overall coherence to mental health services.
- The care trust model would be a natural next step in the longstanding working relationship between local health and social care services. In particular, integrating services within one organisation with a single strategy and vision for the service, supported by a single management structure, would demonstrate the genuine and strong commitment of local partners to work in a unified and consistent way to shape the future of mental health services in Sandwell.
- A care trust would help to overcome a number of practical difficulties with previous arrangements (such as staff being employed by different organisations and therefore having different terms and conditions of employment; different agencies having different policies, approaches and priorities; different governance arrangements and accountability streams; the risk of duplication etc.).
- The care trust model includes nominated local authority members on the care trust board as non-executives, extending the role of local government within health and offering a level of local accountability that cannot be achieved through Health Act flexibilities. Shared accountability arrangements are also ensured through the role of the mental health partnership board as single commissioners of services, representing and speaking for host organisations.

Essential preconditions

In developing proposals for the future of mental health services, there have been a number of key preconditions which have facilitated partnership working.

Leadership

There are a large number of factors that have contributed to the success of the partnership arrangements in Sandwell, not least that they have not happened overnight and that key players have actively managed their emerging and on-going relationships. These leaders have often been crucial to shaping the services in Sandwell and individuals have been described as having a certain 'personal chemistry' (Martin, 2002, p 26) that appears to be firmly built on mutual trust and the shared sense of direction suggested by Hunter (2000) as crucial to sustainability. This has been reinforced by explicit statements of partnership based on a number of shared ground rules of behaviour (which are often identified within the literature as indicators of successful partnership). These include:

- planning together
- reducing territorialism
- sharing information
- agreeing to differ
- being flexible
- agreeing standards and values
- understanding each other.

The culture in Sandwell that has developed from this high level of co-operation and single approach has placed it in an advantageous position on a number of occasions to consider and implement new ideas and ways of working. In turn, the notion that strategy can no longer be driven by single agencies has become embedded within the local planning and delivery framework. Significant progress in developing relationships beyond the usual health and social services boundary to include education, housing and leisure have fortunately been acknowledged by the designation of Sandwell as an HAZ in 1998. Indeed Martin (2002) suggests that this joined up thinking across agencies and interests has become intrinsic to local working and is no longer seen as a 'bolt on'.

Some of this success results from focusing on a common vision for provision rather than on structures, which Poxton (2001) has identified as serving only to dominate the agenda and distract from the real changes in culture that are required to successfully deliver joined up working (*see* Chapter 1).

Learning and preparation

In creating an environment where joint working is the norm, there is a high expectation that we will find solutions together. This has led to a richness of learning that has evolved from both the successful and less successful ventures and that now serves to influence the overall strategy for services and assist in identifying risks and consequent contingency planning. In many instances, new schemes and developments have been built on those already in place.

Early informal and formal discussion about how changes could be made to achieve and deliver the NSF, focusing on the patient/client pathway, proved to be invaluable in assisting key partners to arrive at a clearer vision for service development and greater integration of mental health services. A theoretical grounding in what was happening nationally, what was working well and what opportunities this presented contributed not only a richness of knowledge and expertise, but also provided a robust challenge to current thinking.

Involving stakeholders

The subsequent journey with stakeholders, which led to the debate around whether a care trust was the right option for Sandwell, provided an opportunity not only for leaders to share their views, but also and more importantly to listen to the users, carers and providers of services. Support from external agencies in facilitating these events and in analysing the data gathered has ensured that the process of arriving at the proposals contained within the consultation was based on sound information. At the same time, it has also been crucial to keep key stakeholders informed both through formal committee papers and through a process of regular updates. This was particularly important for the local authority, giving assurance not only about the process being undertaken but also allowing debate to take place regarding the implications of the Care Trust being an NHS body. This has provided an important opportunity not only for local authority members to influence the configuration of the Board and, in so doing, ensure that the knowledge of the council and its affairs are brought to Care Trust meetings as appropriate, but also to gain members' confidence and support for the service development.

Involvement with unions and staff

Staff representatives and unions have been involved in the planning and implementation of the Care Trust from an early stage, and as active members of the project board have made significant contributions to all issues relating to staff. The different cultures and approaches of local authority and health staff representatives and unions have proved to be challenging whilst very productive and have resulted in effective inter-organisational relationships that previously did not exist and which will have direct benefits for staff in the future.

Project management

The required capacity and dedicated project management were initially underestimated at the beginning of the project, resulting in slow and frustrating progress. Lack of progress in appointment led to key directors or managers managing the project without sufficient capacity. The conclusion reached has been that dedicated project management time and skills are essential for successful delivery within tight timescales.

Emerging themes and issues

While it is too early to predict the full implications of establishing a care trust, a number of early themes and issues have begun to emerge.

Terms and conditions and pay differentials

Differences in pay structures have emerged in developing the new structures. It appears that, generally, the NHS currently has lower rates of pay than social services, particularly at the level of healthcare support workers and community care officers. This has not always been the case, but it is likely that these differences between organisational pay structures, where staff are working side by side on different terms and conditions, will continue and will have implications for recruitment and retention in the future. Any attempts at a harmonisation agenda will therefore need to be managed in such a way as to minimise the legal employment implications. The effects of single status and equal pay being pursued by council staff are likely to have financial implications for staff transferring to the Care Trust and will therefore need to be addressed within the partnership agreement.

Recent clarity around options for transfer/retention of pension schemes has been long awaited and much welcomed, although the practicalities of actually offering choices to staff have been devolved to the local level and the process for admission agreements has been laborious and prolonged.

Organisational development

The process of formal consultation created a period of limbo, during which planning implementation became somewhat static or frustratingly limited. Then, all of a sudden, expectations for preparatory implementation were expected to take place and suddenly time was beginning to run out. The need to manage this process to ensure both good communication and that the essential components of an organisational development programme are identified and started cannot be underestimated. Many opportunities can be lost during this preparation phase and ownership of the agenda has been crucial as the move towards greater integration begins to take place. The mechanics of moving into a single organisation and developing an appropriate organisational development programme for this, whilst at the same time maintaining the partnership relationship, requires careful balance. In addition, many staff have worked in the borough for several years and there is a strong local culture of loyalty and service to both organisations, which will need to be fostered and nurtured if staff are to be fully informed and engaged in the changes taking place.

Change management

As with all complex organisational changes, it would also be unrealistic to expect everyone to be fully committed to changing the way in which they work. There are still groups of staff and individuals who, for whatever reason, find it difficult either to share the vision or to make some of the changes required, resulting in mistrust, deep suspicion or lack of co-operation. The focus directed on changing the way in which services are delivered in order to deliver the NSF agenda has been helpful in engaging staff, service users and carers, but cannot be at the risk of ignoring the individual. Managers will need to be mindful to manage this change process in an active manner.

Evaluation

BCMHT and Social Inclusion and Health are committed to undertaking a longitudinal study of the emergence and implementation of the Care Trust through the Institute for Health and Social Care Policy at King's College, London and the Health Services Management Centre, University of Birmingham. This will provide an opportunity to explore the organisational challenges presented by care trust status and to try something different without being preoccupied with structures. Early discussion regarding care trusts identified better outcomes for service users and carers as fundamental to any judgement of their success and it is therefore appropriate that service users and carers are an intrinsic component of the current evaluation process.

Governance and accountability

With new arrangements for dual accountability to the local authority and the NHS, greater clarity and shared understanding will need to be achieved around the statutory responsibilities at all levels within the Care Trust, with no blurring or gaps. Through governance arrangements, local agreement has been reached to ensure up to three nominated council members sit as non-executive members of the Board to reflect the diversity of local needs. Their role and responsibility as paid members of the Board will no doubt present challenges (as they bring their knowledge of the council rather than representation) and a code of conduct will need to be agreed which provides a framework for reconciling diverse and potentially conflicting interests.

The partnership Board is still in its infancy and its relationship with the local implementation team and individual providers is yet to develop. As the single commissioning arm for local mental health services, it plays a vital part in assuring governance and accountability and working with providers to develop the shared strategy.

How do we move on?

An incremental approach to more integrated working has now afforded an opportunity to build on what has been developed so far, particularly in extending a more social model of dis(ability) and rehabilitation as partners begin to look at children's and older people's services to examine the options for their future and how services can be changed to make them more effective. This dynamic engages a wider range of players and consequently opens up further debate on our partnership and sustainability.

Conclusion

As the Sandwell Mental Health and Social Care NHS Trust went 'live' in April 2003, partners were confident that the history of partnership working which Sandwell enjoys will help the local health and social care community rise to the challenges that the new Care Trust is likely to create. However, the creation of the Care Trust has only been made possible by a number of local characteristics, which may not necessarily be present in other areas of the country. Chief amongst these are:

• a history of joint working and a desire to develop more integrated health and social services
• a commitment to partnership working that is based on personalities, close relationships, leadership, trust and mutual understanding rather than on formal structures.

Against this background, establishing a care trust is not a new or a structural issue at all, but rather a logical next step on the road to closer partnership working in Sandwell.

References

Black Country Mental Health Trust (2002) *Black Country Mental Health Trust Annual Report 2002*. LG Davis, Birmingham.

Department of Health (1999) *National Service Framework for Mental Health*. DoH, London.

Department of Health (2001a) *Shifting the Balance of Power within the NHS: securing delivery*. DoH, London.

Department of Health (2001b) *Valuing People: a new strategy for learning disability for the 21st century*. TSO, London.

Hunter D (2000) Pitfalls of arranged marriages. *Health Service J*. 23 November: 22–3.

Martin D (2002) The Sandwell Partnership. *Managing Community Care*. **10**(2): 26.

Poxton R (2001) *Health and Social Care Partnership Working: towards integration*. Institute for Applied Health and Social Policy, King's College, London.

CHAPTER 10

The Hampshire experience

Terry Butler and Angela Jeffrey

The Hampshire experience outlined in this chapter illustrates the ambivalence with which local managers, members and practitioners view the government's care trust 'experiments'. On the one hand, there is a passion locally for creating a seamless service for the recipients of health and social care, coupled with the determination that across local government and health overstretched resources are used to maximum effect through integrated working. On the other hand, there remains both a strong scepticism that a new single organisation and legal entity accountable to the Secretary of State can better fulfil local aspirations or that the organisational turmoil required to become a care trust will achieve desired outcomes (of better services).

Hampshire's early experience of care trusts (and of partnership working more generally) clearly points to two conclusions. First, that creating more accessible, flexible and responsive services across health and social care can be achieved relatively quickly and painlessly without major organisational disruption. Second, that partnership working across the statutory and independent sectors is more likely to be enhanced by an approach which combines development with consolidation rather than being preoccupied with the radical reshaping of organisational structures, accountabilities and support arrangements.

The local government context

The initiative to participate as a care trust pilot was 'sparked off' in Hampshire County Council Social Services Department as it was embarking on a remodelling of its services in early 2001 (Hampshire County Council, 2001). The publication of *The NHS Plan* (DoH, 2000), the roll out of a number of government NSFs (DoH, 1998, 1999, 2001a, b) and growing concerns as to whether resources (both human and financial) were being consistently deployed to best effect led the Director of Social Services to believe that significant internal management changes were required. His Department had last been reorganised in 1997 as one of the consequences of the imposition of local government reorganisation, which created two new unitary authorities (Portsmouth and Southampton) from cities that had previously formed part of Hampshire. Although this reorganisation had brought a number of adverse consequences for the Department, the opportunity had been taken to achieve closer working with the district councils in 'continuing Hampshire' (population 1.2 m). Nowhere was this more promising than with New Forest District Council (population 170 000) where relationships between officers/ members of the district and county councils and partnership working with the voluntary sector were all very strong.

The 2001/02 remodelling of the Social Services Department was designed to achieve three principal aims.

- **The delivery of better services across all client groups** (children and families, older people, people with learning disabilities, people with physical impairments, and those with mental health problems) both to satisfy the requirements of the government's NSFs (with the accompanying regime of monitoring, scrutiny and league tables) and to pursue related local aspirations (particularly the empowerment of service users and carers, building on the Department's already strong position, in particular in offering direct payments and family group conferences).
- **The more consistent control and deployment of resources**: staff, finance and capital assets. The strongest criticism in an otherwise complimentary report of the Audit Commission/Social Services Inspectorate's Joint Review of Hampshire in 1999 was the lack of consistency of investment and standards of service provision across the county. This, coupled with differential performance of budget management across seven area teams, suggested improvements were required.
- **Integrated working with health**. There was a strong recognition within the department that integration was 'the only game in town', especially for services to adults and older people. This was backed by encouragement from members and the leader of the county council, who felt that irrespective of the fact that the county council was strongly Conservative it wished to 'work with the Labour government' and would not 'play politics with people's lives'.

This enabled the Director of Social Services and Executive Cabinet Member for social care to pursue a mission of strengthening links with the emerging StHA for Hampshire and the Isle of Wight and the seven PCTs across the county. The most tangible manifestation of that mission was the establishment of eight senior partnership manager posts to act as a bridge between local government and the various new health bodies in Hampshire.

Therefore, between July 2001 and September 2002, the Social Services Department was reorganised to establish the county-wide specialist management of client groups and a matrix of formal county-wide and local partnership arrangements with health (*see* Figure 10.1).

Motives

Initially, Hampshire decided to 'register' as a national care trust pilot (although the actual process and what this might entail was extremely unclear at the time). From the beginning, this decision was taken by the key partners (the county council, the New Forest PCT and New Forest District Council) as much because of our collective desire to influence government thinking and shape national policies

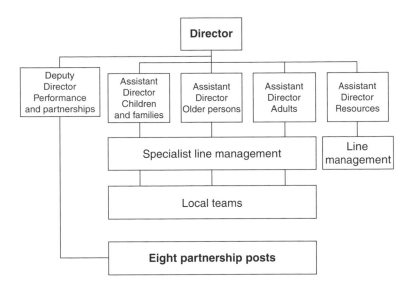

Figure 10.1   New management arrangements.

as because of a belief that we were climbing on a fast track to becoming a care trust. We particularly wanted to explore with colleagues nationally the alternative models of governance and make a reality of the active engagement of and account-ability to local citizens. We were (and still are) also keen to learn from others and take advantage of any resources the government might make available to us preferentially as a pilot site. Our registration as a pilot was viewed as one of a number of initiatives across the county to pursue integrated working, others being the exploration of using the Health Act 1999 flexibilities (*see* Chapter 2), establishing a partnership approach with the StHA to Health Scrutiny and setting up more effective arrangements between education, health and social services for helping children and young people with severe disabilities or behavioural problems. We were not anticipating, and did not enjoy, an easy ride!

The NHS context

At the same time as the local government context described above was develop-ing, the health service was also reorganising. New PCTs were either in place or evolving across Hampshire. The New Forest PCT had, from its creation in April 2001 (and prior to that in its application and development phase) recognised that it had a unique opportunity to design an organisation which would deliver health and social care in partnership for the population of the New Forest. The publi-cation of *The NHS Plan* in July 2000 underpinned our local vision for modernising the NHS for the New Forest. In particular, we wanted to build on our track record of joint working to meet the needs of the local population, not simply in the context of health and health improvement, but also in the wider context of social care and the environment.

The PCT is co-terminous with New Forest District Council and an area of Hampshire County Council Social Services. This, coupled with a significant provider role for the PCT with five community hospitals and a small acute unit at Lymington (together with four acute trust providers from whom it commissions healthcare), has given the PCT a unique opportunity to create a genuinely new organisation. It aims, as far as possible, to remove any traditional barriers that have previously existed and impeded service improvements to the people of the New Forest who need access to health and social care.

Shortly after its inception in the summer of 2001, a further opportunity to take our vision forward was afforded to us in considering the opportunity of care trust status. This opportunity came at a time when the PCT was still getting to grips with the scale of the change it needed to address and with understanding its inheritance. Whilst being keen to pursue the care trust approach, the New Forest PCT did not pursue it at that time for the following reasons:

- the risk that a new organisation would catapult us forward into yet more change and change fatigue
- a difficult financial position with a deficit to manage
- the danger of going too far too soon
- the need to take our constituents and partners with us.

Since 2001, moreover, a range of additional responsibilities have been added to the PCT's portfolio as a result of the demise of health authorities, the creation of StHAs and additional functions that needed to be undertaken by the PCT. These include:

- assessing health needs
- commissioning healthcare for its registered population
- provision of a range of healthcare services
- developing and supporting primary care
- working in partnership with other local statutory and voluntary organisations
- encouraging and developing community involvement and input into service provision.

Early experiences

In February 2002, a multi-agency workshop was held in the New Forest with the theme of 'Developing Partnerships'. The workshop focused on two topics: 'Fears, aspirations, hopes and concerns' and 'Moving forward for service users' (*see* Boxes 10.1 and 10.2 for key themes).

Box 10.1 Examples of key concerns about partnership working

Personnel
- accountability and management
- loss of professional management
- loss of specialist skills
- fears of assimilation, being squeezed out
- lack of understanding about each other's roles

- different HR policies: job security, differences in terms and conditions of service and contractual changes.

Estates
- co-location – ideal but is it realistic?

Finance
- budget constraints
- charging policies
- pooled budgets – maintenance in the context of potential draining of resources to acute services and impact on other services.

Organisational development
- fear of the unknown/change
- speed of constant change
- expectations too high
- commitment and involvement of GPs
- finding time to develop
- communication with staff and users
- local ownership
- politics and unpredictability of government policy.

Organisational cultural differences
- medical versus social model (fear from users of less holistic view).

Box 10.2   Key aspirations: examples

Personnel
- improved recruitment
- learning about each other's roles and responsibilities
- training for new roles – about doing a different role, learning new skills
- opportunities for joint training.

Making partnership a positive option for staff as well as users
- increased attractiveness of job
- multi-tasking of workforce.

Finance
- greater equity of service provision
- work towards pooled budget
- freeing up resources – which can be used to tackle need elsewhere
- better/more efficient use of resources
- stop arguing about who pays
- developing brokerage and advocacy.

Organisational development
- being able to develop as a site of excellence
- we direct change
- build on existing expertise and momentum
- understanding of other agencies' strengths and constraints
- culture change
- clearer and simpler access to services
- agree protocols
- build sustainable partnerships, structures and services
- linked planning
- continuity of care
- holistic approach to integrated services
- navigator one-stop shops – seamless service
- less paperwork
- integrated monitoring and evaluation.

This diverse range of issues and concerns gave us an early indication that achieving care trust status was an extremely challenging option and underlined the view that our focus should be on achieving better outcomes with and for users. As a result, 'moving forward' was seen as concentrating on the practicality of:

Personnel

- Joint training, shadowing, joint care competencies and joint moving and handling training.
- Flexible working.

Estates

- One-stop shops.
- Base for integrated rapid response team.

Finance

- All agencies and government to put cash into joint budget.

Organisational development

- Protocols: all working under the same guidelines.
- Improving contacts.
- Awareness of each others' roles, responsibilities, remit and boundaries.
- Improving transport and local services.
- Developing night sitting service.
- Ensuring GPs are involved.

- Single assessment process put in place.
- De-jargonise communication.
- Confidentiality:
  – share at agreed levels
  – improved joint ownership of information
  – joint notes or using each others' client held notes.

Projects

- Joint funded projects (such as care and repair, training).
- Effective development of generic/specialist floating support service for those outside criteria for statutory services.
- Streamlined joint sensory impairment service.
- Mapping care pathways (i.e. for stroke).
- New Lymington Hospital (*see below*).

Staff and user involvement

- Users and staff are involved in determining where to integrate.

As we embarked on the next 12 months of joint working we were constantly reminded of Leutz's (1999) five laws of integration:

- you can integrate all of the services for some of the people, or some of the services for all of the people, but you can't integrate all of the services for all of the people
- integration costs before it pays
- your integration is my fragmentation
- you can't integrate a square peg and a round hole
- s/he who integrates, calls the tune.

These laws seemed to us to suggest that we should be cautious in selecting our areas for integration, but rigorous in pursuing those that we did select.

Tangible progress

To date, the most significant areas of tangible progress relate to services for older people and examples include the following:

Lymington Infirmary

This major initiative during 2002/03 relates to the reprovision of 37 beds from an old workhouse/rehabilitation hospital in Lymington to other sites within the community. The proposals have been worked up jointly with health and social care, and consulted upon with the local community on a joint basis. The aim of reproviding the inpatient services delivered at Lymington Infirmary is to address environmental issues there, whilst maintaining and enhancing the range of locally accessible services for people in the New Forest. The main elements of the proposal were to reprovide inpatient services by two methods.

- **Developing multi-disciplinary multi-agency locality teams**: The proposal is to develop up to five multi-disciplinary locality teams which provide a range of health and social care services to older people in the New Forest. The core teams will include district and rehabilitation nurses, home carers, medical staff, occupational therapists, physiotherapists, social workers and secretarial support. There will also be access to other specialist services, such as a dietician, a speech and language therapist, a stroke co-ordinator and specialist nurses.
- **Improving opportunities for 'intermediate care'**: Discussions between the PCT and the county council indicate that, with the refurbishment of Solent Mead (a local authority care home) in Lymington, there will be four beds available for intermediate care. These beds will be allocated to patients who meet the agreed criteria. Discussions continue regarding this and similar provision elsewhere in the New Forest. These beds will be supported by community nursing and locality rehabilitation teams.

Rapid response teams

This is a new joint initiative developed in 2002 between the PCT and social services to prevent hospital admissions and allow the support of complex discharges in the community. It is proving a very successful initiative. The aim is to provide patients and their families with short-term support as it is needed to promote a return to independent living. Trained staff visit patients at home and agree an assessment of their needs. The team can also arrange long-term care where appropriate.

Care managers in GP practices

Another joint initiative between the PCT and social services is the attachment of care managers to primary healthcare teams. This has been a gradual and ongoing development over the past few years and we are now pursuing a more comprehensive and pro-active approach. All practices within the PCT have been divided into zones to provide a local focus. This approach has had a very positive response as it has a variety of benefits which include avoiding duplication, more effective use of resources, easier access for users and carers, better co-ordination of health and social care and earlier response to avoid deterioration. Plans are now underway to broaden the scheme and promote user/carer involvement.

Delayed transfers of care

By working in partnership we have managed to reduce the number of patients currently occupying a hospital bed whilst waiting for more appropriate care by more than two thirds. There has been a focus on working together and ensuring excellent communication. Social services staff have provided the ward managers and senior nurses in our hospitals with training and access to information. Our approach includes bed management meetings held each week between health and social care to identify any potential problems and ensure planning can start as soon as possible to resolve them. During 2002/03, social services have been allocated money through the government's 'Cash for Change' grant, which has funded prompt access to nursing and residential home care. A home care direct service facilitates timely discharges from hospital, prevents unnecessary admissions and provides increased home care for New Forest clients. The PCT has also funded a lead nurse with special responsibility for delayed transfers of care and NHS funded nursing in nursing homes. Progress has been carefully monitored through collation of data to ensure delayed transfers stay at reduced levels. When the going gets tough the numbers of delayed transfers begin to rise again and this does test the strength of our partnerships!

Home treatment team

This is another initiative developed jointly between the PCT and social services and is the first of its kind in the area. It aims to fast-track patients from hospital beds to the comfort of their own homes by providing a team of health and social care professionals to deliver services at home. The scheme has proved popular with patients and successful in taking pressure off the heavily burdened orthopaedic departments of our local hospitals. Plans are now underway to spread the scheme to other parts of the New Forest.

Single assessment process

The PCT is working in partnership with social services and West Hampshire Trust to implement the single assessment process within the New Forest. The single assessment process underpins joint working, helping to ensure a more standardised and holistic assessment of older people's needs and minimise duplication to ensure better use of operational staff's time. Single assessment will also assist in information sharing between professions in order that care can be provided promptly and tailored to meet older people's needs. The PCT has appointed a part time project lead for the single assessment process, who is responsible for working across the agencies to progress the project.

Conclusions: next steps

The progress of a number of joint working initiatives in the New Forest area shows that, with agencies working closely together, local services can be improved and more efficient use made of resources. Towards the end of 2002 we formally reviewed progress again and determined not to push for going live as a care trust in April 2003, but to hold this as an option at a later stage. The principal reasons for that decision were:

- there is still much to do in achieving a common understanding of the respective roles, strengths and constraints across partner agencies

- there would be a disproportionate amount of work over a very short time scale to reach the April 2003 starting date
- the creation of a care trust would involve the disaggregation of several key aspects of the county council's financial and personnel support arrangements where the balance of costs and benefits remain questionable
- much progress has been made on integrating the line management of services to improve outcomes for users/patients without the need for a totally separate organisation.

From both the county council and PCT's perspective, the deployment of the new partnership managers is proving invaluable in pushing out the boundaries of joint working. Across the county, they sit on all PCT executive committees. Based on the particularly successful role of the partnership manager for the New Forest PCT, the county council and PCT have agreed that the partnership manager post will now become Deputy PCT Chief Executive with the key responsibility for the integration of health and social care at a very senior level in both organisations. This post is a joint appointment currently being advertised between New Forest PCT and Hampshire County Council Social Services Department. The key responsibilities of this jointly funded post are to lead the way forward for the integration of health and social care services in the New Forest. This underpins the strategic direction agreed by both organisations to pursue integration of services rather than the care trust model. The role of the postholder, in this phase of the partnership development, will be an enabling one, determining the direction of travel towards integration within an agreed vision and strategy. Their key tasks will include:

- leading the development of integrated approaches to health and social care
- the development of integrated approaches to organisational development and HR across the two organisations
- developing an integrated approach to performance management
- playing a full part in the corporate approach to developing the vision and strategy for both organisations leading to integration.

Whilst further government guidance on the role of local councillors in relation to overview and scrutiny of healthcare is eagerly awaited, each PCT has an elected county council member attending its board meeting as an observer. Alongside the joint work on scrutiny with the StHA and frequent dialogue between board chairs and the executive member for social care, this is proving successful in developing a common understanding of the nature of our joint challenges and opportunities.

Overall, therefore, our recent experience suggests that care trusts are not the right solution for us in Hampshire at this point in time and we have chosen other routes to achieve the closer integration of health and social care.

References

Department of Health (1998) *Quality Protects: transforming children's services*. DoH, London.

Department of Health (1999) *National Service Framework for Mental Health*. DoH, London.

Department of Health (2000) *The NHS Plan: a plan for investment, a plan for reform.* TSO, London.

Department of Health (2001a) *National Service Framework for Older People.* DoH, London.

Department of Health (2001b) *Valuing People: a new strategy for learning disability for the 21st century.* TSO, London.

Hampshire County Council (2001) *Rising to the Challenge: improving health and social care in Hampshire – report to Social Services Committee, 23 March 2001.* Hampshire County Council.

Leutz W (1999) Five laws for integrating medical and social services: lessons from the US and UK. *Milbank Quarterly.* **77**(1): 77–110.

CHAPTER 11

Care trusts: emerging themes and issues

Edward Peck and Jon Glasby

The policy context

In reflecting on progress in the development of health and social care partnerships since 1997, it is important not to lose a sense of history. By the mid-1990s, joint planning was largely discredited (*see*, for example, Hudson and Henwood, 2002; Nocon, 1994), joint commissioning was hindered by financial regulations (Audit Commission/CMHSD, 1997) and a Labour Opposition spokesperson could resign partly over the reluctance of the party to countenance change in the structural relationships between the NHS and social services. Indeed, New Labour policy under Frank Dobson, its first Secretary of State, whilst famously proclaiming its commitment to 'bringing down the Berlin Wall', continued to be wary of innovations in structure (DoH, 1998).

It was by no means inevitable, therefore, that by 2003 elements of health and social services would have merged into care trusts in seven localities around the UK. Additional sites are in the pipeline, as are the first tranche of children's trusts, and in some local authorities social services departments have disappeared altogether, leaving only a nominated officer somewhere in the local authority with the specific residual duties spelt out by the Chief Inspector. Furthermore, these care trusts represent only the tip of the iceberg of partnership initiatives around the UK. So what happened? Why did the inertia and caution of the mid-1990s turn into the major organisational and service change evident by 2003, apparently resisted only in a small number of localities?

Summarising the argument in Chapter 1 by Poxton, a number of factors can be identified. Much has been made of New Labour's commitment to 'joined-up government' (6 *et al.*, 2002) made manifest early in its first term by the creation of action zones in health, education and employment. This commitment was itself an aspect of the party's endorsement of the theories of new public management, where, by the final years of the old century, the adoption of networks were seen as a 'third way' alternative to the allegedly failed ideologies of hierarchy (typical of the 1980s) and markets (common in the 1990s). At the same time, reported failures in the co-ordination of public services (from Christopher Clunis to Victoria Climbié) provided stark evidence of the price of agencies failing to work in partnership. Simultaneously, one or two localities seemed to show the way forward through innovations which both anticipated policy and gave government examples of good practice with which to illustrate that policy. As the enthusiasm for enhanced partnership spread amongst ministers and civil servants, local government, and more specifically social services departments and social workers, seemed unable to articulate a compelling case for social care not being brought closer to, and in the example of care trusts ultimately merged into, the NHS. Arguably, this was not for want of potential ammunition, as Chapter 7 by Hudson ably demonstrates (and Hudson is undoubtedly one of the 'commentators' referred to by Giles in Chapter 6).

Much has been written in the literature on organisational change about the tendency of organisations in the same field to copy each other's innovations. In the case of partnership working between health and social care, the impact of the early adopters, such as Somerset, was undoubtedly important. In addition, it is certainly true that many managers involved in early onset partnerships saw genuine benefits that they wanted to pursue further; it can be no co-incidence that the six of the seven care trusts established by April 2003 were in localities which possessed HAZs. Glendinning and colleagues, in Chapter 2, report remarkable consistency amongst the managers that her team interviewed about the advantages that will flow from application of the Health Act 1999 flexibilities. There are also clear similarities in the accounts of their local innovations provided by O'Leary and Macfarlane (*see* Chapters 8 and 9). Clearly, a new consensus had rapidly emerged in the system about the virtues of health and social care partnership.

Nonetheless, this tendency towards replication and consensus was encouraged by a government that was taking an increasingly active interest in the implementation of its policy. Although they reluctantly backed away from the power to impose care trusts that they had trailed in *The NHS Plan* (DoH, 2000), ministers and civil servants took a number of other steps to ensure that managers pursued partnership arrangements (e.g. drug action teams were only to be allowed to access government resources if they could demonstrate that they would commission services through a pooled budget). Poxton raises other examples in his chapter. More recently, an application made by two mental health trusts to merge seems to have been approved by ministers only on the condition that a care trust is created in due course (personal communication, *see below* for further discussion).

The government's strategy was not all about sticks, however. Immediately following its creation, the Chief Executive of the Somerset Partnerships Trust was feted by government: he was the keynote speaker at a major national DoH conference on leadership, invited to join the National Mental Health Task Force and asked to attend a briefing meeting with the Prime Minister (which was cancelled due to the arrival of baby Leo, but replaced by an invitation to a reception at 10 Downing Street 12 months later). The message was simple: the integration of health and social care was viewed positively by the government and would be rewarded. The carrots have continued, albeit in a more modest form, for example the financial support offered by the DoH to pilot children's trusts (*see below* and DoH, 2002).

But why, if managers were so keen to pursue partnership, did the government feel it necessary to apply the sticks and the carrots described above? Two factors seem to explain the paradox. The first is the different meaning ascribed to time by managers and politicians. For the former group, three years may seem a short period within which to build the personal and organisational relationships, particularly at a time of constant structural change in the NHS, which are required to underpin effective partnerships. To the latter, three years may be a ministerial lifetime where failure to produce tangible outcomes can be easily construed as local inertia.

The second factor relates more prosaically to the 'notification' process put in place by the DoH. This required that it must be notified of any uses of the flexibilities under the Health Act. However, as no apparent benefits to localities followed notification, many simply did not bother and, consequently, the uptake seemed paltry. In 2002, when it went out to actively seek information about their use, the DoH was able to double the amount of money in the system that it could report to ministers was being handled through application of the flexibilities. Furthermore, of course, many of the partnership arrangements being put in place simply went under the DoH's radar as they did not involve Health Act flexibilities (for example, Somerset's commissioning approach relied on parallel, not pooled, budgets and thus did not require notification).

Nonetheless, it is also important to note that the government has never pinned its political credibility on the number of care trusts, in comparison with the importance to Kenneth Clarke in 1991 of having a significant number of 'first wave' NHS trusts (or perhaps to Alan Milburn or John Reid of having a goodly number of foundation hospitals). Despite the sticks and the carrots, care trusts are not central to ministers' concerns. This slightly marginal position has both benefits and weaknesses. It means that care trusts can typically be seen as an option that localities can choose to pursue and are not something that are going to be routinely enforced. At the same time, it means that their pursuance means having to make sense of policy – especially health policy – that may not have been drafted with merged health and social care organisations in mind. The best recent example is the NHS initiative known as 'Agenda for Change'.

The lack of consistency between the terms and conditions for health and social care staff within care trusts has been a major issue both in the debate over their desirability and in the objectives set by the boards of the initial adopters. At an early stage, the DoH attempted to undertake some national work on harmonisation of these terms and conditions, but this has since gone relatively quiet and the creation of care trusts went ahead with the issue still outstanding. Subsequently, 'Agenda for Change' has proposed a limited number of pay bands which will bring together into one framework most of the disparate tasks undertaken by NHS personnel, which are currently covered by a myriad of national agreements. This would have been an opportunity to reconcile the financial rewards attaching to social care activities undertaken within care trusts to those of traditional NHS staff. Unfortunately, this opportunity appears to have been missed and care trusts will have to continue to deal with the impact of the apparent inequities, and attempt to resolve them, by themselves.

Further, it is becoming apparent that some of the guidance issued by the DoH is not always dealing with the complexities that local implementation is throwing up. For example, a recent national event on care trust governance in May 2003 suggested that the seven existing care trusts at this time were all struggling to a greater or lesser extent with issues such as (Glasby *et al.*, 2003):

- the precise role of local authority nominees (who are representatives of their local authorities, but also board members with wider corporate responsibilities) on care trust boards
- the role of users and carers on care trust boards

- the future role of social services departments if a number of adult services are delegated to care trusts
- future relationships with the wider local authority and, for provider-based care trusts, primary care.

The impact of constant reorganisation

If primary care-based care trusts are finding the relationship with local authority members uncomfortable on occasions, the secondary care-based ones are struggling with the change in local context represented by the advent of PCTs. As many of the chapters of this book argue, context is crucial to the creation of partnerships and central to context are characters and co-terminosity. In the case of the first five mental healthcare trusts, both are potentially challenged by the emergence of PCTs.

The partnerships which underpinned the development of these five care trusts relied to a greater or lesser extent on the support of the health authorities abolished in 2002 (it is surely no coincidence that these five care trusts have the organisational boundaries of the health authorities in existence immediately prior to the implementation of *Shifting the Balance of Power Within the NHS*) and their relationship with the local authority. These health authorities possessed the commonality of boundaries with one or more local authorities upon which personal and organisational relationships could be built. Many of the roles of these health authorities have now been taken over by at least two and usually more PCTs covering the same geographical patch and often led by managers new to the local scene and understandably keen to assert their authority and independence. One of the major implications of these changes in characters and co-terminosity has been for joint commissioning and partnership boards where the approach of the health authority established with the local authority has not necessarily been replicated by the PCTs, and this has introduced unwelcome uncertainty into the lives of the care trusts.

At the same time, the development of PCGs into PCTs between 1998 and 2002 has meant the sort of internal instability that has undoubtedly contributed to the small number of primary-based care trusts to date. The newness of the New Forest PCT in 2001 was a key influence, Butler and Jeffrey point out in Chapter 10, for not pursuing care trust status in this part of Hampshire. As they argue, the lack of this formal structural innovation does not mean that primary care and social care have not being growing their relationship – witness the number of joint directors of public health appointed since April 2002 – but there is much less history of common ground between general practice and social work than there is between psychiatry and social work. Nor is the current configuration of PCTs sacrosanct, and although formal mergers look unlikely this side of the 2004/05 election, many are exploring ways of gaining more commissioning leverage on acute providers through various means of collaboration with their neighbours (Smith *et al.*, 2002). As a consequence, the prospects of large numbers of primary-care based care trusts coming forward in the near future seems remote.

Of course, six years of hyperactive New Labour policy making in relation to health and social care should have meant that such changes in context were to be expected and there is no reason why care trusts should expect to be immune. The latest partnership vehicle suggested by the government – children's trusts – has been prompted by the government's impatience with the quality of services for children provided by the education departments of local authorities as well as social services. Located within local government, this new initiative raises a number of questions, such as (Glasby, 2003):

- how to extend traditional health and social care partnerships to include education
- how to establish appropriate links with acute healthcare and wider children and young people's initiatives such as Connexions or youth offending teams
- whether or not children's trusts will commission or provide services (or both)
- whether they will be based on co-located and integrated teams or whether they will be virtual organisations based on firmer links between existing organisations
- where child protection sits in relation to children's trusts.

Organisational culture and development

One of the central messages about care trusts that is also going to be important to the effectiveness of children's trusts relates to the importance of 'culture'. Much of the perceived difference between health and social care organisations, and the professionals within them, is expressed in terms of disparities in 'culture' (a point stressed in the chapters about Somerset and intermediate care in this book). Much has been written about this topic in recent years (e.g. Peck and Crawford, 2002; Peck *et al.*, 2001), not least that the notion of 'culture' within an organisational context is problematic and has many varied definitions. Nonetheless, the definition of Schein (1997) that organisational culture can be thought of as the shared basic assumptions that an organisation or profession learns as it solves problems of adaptation and integration seems to reflect much of the way in which it is used in debates about partnership.

Most of the airport departure lounge literature on culture – the 'culture cookbooks' such as Deal and Kennedy (1982) – assumes that culture can be manipulated by managers for predictable ends. However, some of the descriptive literature on culture challenges this view. For example, Meyerson and Martin (1987) present a schema of three views of culture and cultural change in the literature which they term 'integration', 'differentiation' and 'ambiguity'. The integration approach views culture as an integrating force, 'the social or normative glue that holds together a potentially diverse group of organisational members' (p 624). In this view, cultural change entails an organisation-wide shift in attitudes or beliefs, usually manipulated by senior managers. This is very much the position assumed in the 'culture cookbooks'.

However, the other two views of culture offer less hope to the would-be manipulators. Differentiation emphasises that culture is composed of a collection of values and beliefs, some of which may be contradictory, held by identifiable and disparate sub-cultures. Cultural change in these circumstances will be localised and incremental and will be influenced by a myriad of factors both within and outside of the organisation.

The notion of ambiguity suggests that manifestations of culture are characterised by complexity where differences in meaning and values may be seen as irreconcilable and 'individuals share some viewpoints, disagree about some, and are ignorant and indifferent to others. Consensus, dissensus and confusion coexist' (p 637). In this view, culture is continually changing as the interpretations made by, and the patterns of connections between, individuals form and re-form. Peck *et al.* (2001) found that these three views of culture were exhibited and interacted in their study of Somerset as discussed above.

Parker (2000) also draws on the work of Meyerson and Martin (1987) in reflecting on the extent to which organisational culture can be manipulated. He comes to two conclusions from his consideration of the literature. The first is that 'cultural management in the sense of creating an enduring set of shared beliefs is impossible' (p 228). On the other hand, he suggests that 'it seems perverse to argue that the "climate", "atmosphere", "personality", or culture of an organisation cannot be consciously altered' (p 229). So the considered position seems to be that some manipulation of culture by managers may be possible, but that the impact may be limited and/or unpredictable.

What is certain is that managers need to consider the cultural dimensions of care trusts as they put together their organisational development programmes. If a care trust is going to be more than just the sum of its component parts, then over time it will need to develop ways of thinking and behaving differently. This may mean that the beliefs, values and principles upon which it is based need to be different. What is in the policy context that might support the development of difference? The following paragraphs highlight some of the influences on the authors as they have worked with the Sandwell Mental Health NHS and Social Care Trust on the development of an organisational development (OD) programme.

Some of the principles underpinning *Valuing People: a new strategy for learning disability for the 21st century* (DoH, 2001b) introduce a different paradigm to government policy which could be used to help shape a care trust. For example 'mainstreaming' and 'person centred planning' (PCP) focus attention on the whole person as a 'citizen'. The underlying aim is to enable someone to live, and actively take part, in the local community. Similar ideas, under the broad rubric of 'recovery', are starting to influence national thinking on mental health services. These policy directions have several potential implications for care trusts:

- making detailed planning for individual service users (i.e. person-centred planning) central to the activity of the care trust rather than broad strategies for large populations of undifferentiated users
- making connections with civic society central to the aspirations of the organisation
- establishing an organisation where users and carers are represented and involved with service delivery at all levels.

Building upon these policy directives, other initiatives start to suggest themselves:

- building community accountability into the care trust from the outset with pro-active engagement with parallel structures, e.g. extended scrutiny approaches
- making the care trust accountable to local users and carers (e.g. by introducing users' panels with similar responsibilities to professional executive committees in PCTs)
- challenging traditional flows of financial control (e.g. by pursuing direct payments)

- exploring ideas of local autonomy, rather than central hierarchy, in organisational design (e.g. self-organising teams)
- operating within a culture that challenges gender, race and age discrimination.

In time, presumably, a three-star care trust could also pursue foundation status and create a new form of organisational accountability, combining the new 'elected' stakeholders of the NHS and the traditional elected members of the local authority. Indeed, it could be argued that the stakeholder boards envisaged for foundation hospitals are just one step further on from the expanded membership of care trust boards – an example of policy evolution in action.

One of the key devices in thinking through these cultural issues may be the undertaking of a cultural audit. What is valued in the organisations merging to form the care trust? What is punished? What do the two organisations admire about each other? What creates suspicion in one about the other? Such an audit might provide a firmer foundation on which to base initiatives to support the creation of a different approach for the care trust.

Finally, the routine tools of organisational development – organisational role analysis, learning sets, team-building opportunities – should not be overlooked in the design of a series of interventions. The balance of interventions will vary from site to site. Some will be short term, for example open space events, and some will be long term, for example the extension of the use of direct payments. However, the importance of using organisational development tools to support the successful creation of care trusts can scarcely be doubted, in particular if care trusts are to avoid the problems identified in private sector mergers.

One of the key tools to changing the culture of the care trust, which is explicit in the previous few paragraphs, is the transformation of the organisation and its staff in its relationship with the users which it serves. The allocation of a place on the trust board to a service user discussed by Diane Brodie in Chapter 5 is an important innovation. However, inevitably, the individual service user will have limited impact as all the research on public and private sector boards stresses that they have a powerful symbolic function, but limited influence on individual organisational decisions (Peck *et al.*, 2002). The importance of the board – and thus the presence of the user on the board – is mostly symbolic, signalling the way in which the organisation intends to do its business and, in this case, the importance it attaches to the presence and views of users in the business of the organisation. The user on the board may feel frustrated by his/her lack of power, as indeed may many other members, but it is perhaps unhelpful to describe this approach using the pejorative term 'tokenistic' as this seems to both impute the motives of the organisation and deny the wider implications of their membership.

A means to an end

This discussion of culture, and the aspiration to change culture, brings us back to a key point about care trusts and all such formal partnership arrangements – that they are a means to ends not an end in themselves. These ends may differ between managers, professionals and users in the same patch, and the means adopted may vary across localities. For instance, it would be a brave commentator that challenged Hampshire on, say, its record on the developments of integrated care for older adults in the New Forest, articulated by Butler and Jeffrey, just because it had not pursued a care trust approach to underpin them. Butler and Jeffrey's chapter also suggests local concern about the danger of subsuming social care values under medical ones within a care trust and history may be on their side; one of the first tasks of one of the editors in his NHS career was to support the dismantling in the mid-1980s of the local psychiatric hospital social work department and the integration of the social workers back into area social services offices partly as it was perceived that they had lost their social care perspective and become too compliant to the medical model!

Furthermore, the chapter on intermediate care by Goodwin and Peet has reminded us that there are partnerships beyond health and social care – with the independent sector for instance – that may take on additional importance over forthcoming years. This may well be more of a priority for PCTs, especially as they take on the management of elective waiting lists, than further structural alignment with social care (although the experience and expertise of social care staff in market making and contract management may prove to be a real benefit to them).

As this book has shown, many localities are pursuing approaches to partnership that emphasise processes and relationships at a local level and which do not require structural change. As Giles has argued in Chapter 6, the government genuinely sees the care trust as only one option amongst many; indeed, the DoH has been active in discouraging applications for care trust status from localities that have little history of effective joint working. Unlike the use of the Health Act flexibilities, the creation of a care trust has to be approved by the Secretary of State in the same way as the proposal for any other NHS trust, giving the DoH considerable leverage over potential applicants.

In these circumstances, the pressure apparently being applied to two merging NHS mental health trusts to form a care trust (discussed above) is probably as puzzling to the civil servants involved as it is to commentators such as ourselves. Presumably the no-star status of the social services department, and the widely acknowledged failure of joint working between health and the local authority in the patch, have exasperated politicians to the point where they feel obliged to use informally the power that was formally denied them by the House of Lords. Perhaps one example of enforced partnership will allow us to test the widely held belief that compulsion will undermine effectiveness. It will also act as a sharp reminder to those other localities which combine poor organisational performance with poor inter-agency collaboration about the potential consequences of not sharpening up their act.

Ultimately, the extent to which the initial furore over care trusts has been justified by the creation of just seven examples is obviously debatable, but it is also arguable that those that have chosen other mechanisms have been at least partly prompted by the lively debate that care trusts have engendered. Care trusts are neither the beginning nor the end of initiatives around health and social care partnership in the UK. They inherit both some baggage and some wisdom from the organisational forms that went before them and, in turn, will bequeath some to those that follow. This book will hopefully play a part in enabling those pursuing care trust status to acquire some of the learning from earlier initiatives in partnership and those implementing subsequent arrangements to benefit from the initial experience of care trusts.

References

Audit Commission/CMHSD (1997) *Caring for Citizens*. Audit Commission/CMHSD, London.

Deal TE and Kennedy AA (1982) *Corporate Cultures: the rites and rituals of corporate life*. Addison Wesley, Reading, Massachusetts.

Department of Health (1998) *Partnership in Action: new opportunities for joint working between health and social services – a discussion document*. DoH, London.

Department of Health (2000) *The NHS Plan: a plan for investment, a plan for reform*. TSO, London.

Department of Health (2001a) *Shifting the Balance of Power: securing delivery*. DoH, London.

Department of Health (2001b) *Valuing People: a new strategy for learning disability for the 21st Century*. TSO, London.

Department of Health (2002) *Children's Trusts*. Available online at www.doh.gov.uk/childrenstrusts (accessed 31/10/2002).

Glasby J (2003) *Coming of Age: the role of children's trusts*. Seminar pack based on Health Services Management Centre seminar, 30 April, University of Birmingham, Birmingham.

Glasby J, Hardacre J and Peck E (2003) *Care Trust Governance: policies, principles and progress*. Briefing paper based on Health Services Management Centre Workshop, York, 8 May. A summary is available online via www.integratedcarenetwork.gov.uk

Hudson B and Henwood M (2002) The NHS and social care: the final countdown? *Policy and Politics*. **30**(2): 153–66.

Meyerson D and Martin J (1987) Cultural change: an integration of three different views. *J Management Studies*. **24**(6): 623–43.

Nocon A (1994) *Collaboration in Community Care in the 1990s*. Business Education Publishers, Sunderland.

Parker M (2000) *Organizational Culture and Identity*. Sage, London.

Peck E and Crawford A (2002) 'You say tomato' … culture as signifier of difference in health and social care. *Mental Health Review*. **7**(2): 23–6.

Peck E, Towell D and Gulliver P (2001) The meanings of 'culture' in health and social care: a case study of the combined trust in Somerset. *J Interprofessional Care*. **15**(4): 319–27.

Peck E, Gulliver P, and Towell D (2002) Governance of partnership between health and social services: the experience in Somerset. *Health and Social Care in the Community*. **10**(5): 331–8.

Schein E (1997) *Organizational Change and Leadership*. Bass, San Francisco.

Smith J, Goodwin N and Peck E (2002) *Report of a Review of Organisational Options for Trafford South Primary Care Trust*. HSMC, University of Birmingham, Birmingham.

6 P, Leat D, Seltzer K *et al.* (2002) *Towards Holistic Governance: the new reform agenda*. Palgrave, Basingstoke.

Index